Increasing Physical Activity

Lifestyle Medicine

Series Editor: James M. Rippe

Professor of Medicine, University of Massachusetts Medical School

Led by James M. Rippe, MD, founder of the Rippe Lifestyle Institute, this series is directed to a broad range of researchers and professionals consisting of topical books with clinical applications in nutrition and health, physical activity, obesity management, and applicable subjects in lifestyle medicine.

Increasing Physical Activity: A Practical Guide, *James M. Rippe*

For more information, please visit: www.routledge.com/Lifestyle-Medicine/book-series/CRCLM

Increasing Physical Activity

A Practical Guide

Edited by

James M. Rippe
Founder and Director, Rippe Lifestyle Institute
Professor of Medicine, University of Massachusetts
Medical School

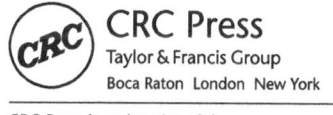

CRC Press
Taylor & Francis Group
Boca Raton London New York

CRC Press is an imprint of the
Taylor & Francis Group, an **informa** business

CRC Press

Boca Raton and London

First edition published 2021

by CRC Press

6000 Broken Sound Parkway NW, Suite 300, Boca Raton, FL 33487-2742

and by CRC Press

2 Park Square, Milton Park, Abingdon, Oxon, OX14 4RN

© 2021 Taylor & Francis Group, LLC

CRC Press is an imprint of Taylor & Francis Group, LLC

Library of Congress Cataloging-in-Publication Data

Names: Rippe, James M., author.
Title: Increasing physical activity : a practical guide / James M. Rippe.
Other titles: Lifestyle medicine series (CRC Press)
Description: First edition. | Boca Raton, FL : CRC Press, 2021. | Series:
Lifestyle medicine series | Includes bibliographical references and
index. | Summary: "The health benefits of regular physical activity are
beyond dispute, yet less than 40% of physicians routinely counsel their
patients on the importance of physical activity. Increasing Physical
Activity: A Practical Guide equips healthcare practitioners to include
physical activity counseling in the daily practice of medicine"--
Provided by publisher.
Identifiers: LCCN 2020029363 (print) | LCCN 2020029364 (ebook) | ISBN
9780367499952 (paperback) | ISBN 9780367500412 (hardback) | ISBN
9781003048589 (ebook)
Subjects: MESH: Exercise | Physical Fitness | Health Promotion--methods |
Healthy Lifestyle | Physician's Role
Classification: LCC RA781 (print) | LCC RA781 (ebook) | NLM QT 256 | DDC
613.7--dc23
LC record available at https://lccn.loc.gov/2020029363
LC ebook record available at https://lccn.loc.gov/2020029364

ISBN: 9780367500412 (hbk)
ISBN: 9780367499952 (pbk)
ISBN: 9781003048589 (ebk)

Typeset in Times
by KnowledgeWorks Global Ltd.

Dedication

To my beautiful wife Stephanie Hart Rippe and our wonderful children Hart, Jaelin, Devon, and Jamie. As Ezra Pound said, "What thou lovest well remains…"

Contents

Preface..ix

Acknowledgments...xv

Author Biography...xvii

Chapter 1   Lifestyle Medicine, Physical Activity, and Health.............................1

Chapter 2   Background and Key Physical Activity Concepts............................15

Chapter 3   Physical Activity and Cardiovascular Disease
Risk-Reduction and Treatment..29

Chapter 4   Physical Activity and the Prevention
and Treatment of Cancer..45

Chapter 5   Physical Activity and Diabetes, Prediabetes, and the
Metabolic Syndrome 57

Chapter 6   Physical Activity in Women's Health..67

Chapter 7   Physical Activity and Youth 79

Chapter 8   Physical Activity in Older Adults..89

Chapter 9   Physical Activity in Individuals with Chronic Conditions..............101

Chapter 10 Physical Activity, Weight Gain, and Obesity 111

Chapter 11 Physical Activity, Cognition, and Brain Health 123

Chapter 12 The Role of Physicians in Promoting and Prescribing
Increased Physical Activity...137

Chapter 13 Exercise Prescription: Practical Applications 153

Chapter 14 Overcoming Sedentary Behavior 165

Chapter 15 Promoting Regular Physical Activity 173

Appendix A 189

Appendix B 193

Appendix C 197

Index 199

Preface

There is no longer any serious doubt that daily habits and actions profoundly impact on short- and long-term health and quality of life. The scientific and medical literature that support this concept are now overwhelming. There are thousands of studies that support the benefits of various aspects of how daily habits and actions impact on health and quality of life.

Though there are many habits and practices that influence health, physical activity is certainly one of the key factors. In fact, if one looks at risk factors both for cardiovascular disease and for all-cause mortality, inactivity is a stronger risk factor for all of these entities than any other single modality. The literature related to physical activity and its health-promoting benefits continues to explode. New studies in this area are published every day. We have been blessed, in the last few years, with the publication of the Physical Activity Guidelines for Americans 2018 Scientific Report. This report is an exhaustive compilation of data that existed up until 2018, related to the various aspects of physical activity and health. This watershed document also provides the basic structure and backbone for the current monograph on Lifestyle Medicine: Physical Activity.

The current volume combines two very important concepts, namely, lifestyle medicine and physical activity, as the title suggests. The overall benefits of a physically active lifestyle are beyond dispute. For example, when inactive individuals are compared to active individuals, the inactive individuals increase their risk of cardiovascular disease between 150% and 240%. A landmark study done a number of years ago from the Centers for Disease Control (CDC) compared individuals who met CDC standards for physical activity with inactive individuals. By the criteria utilized in this study, 80% of individuals in the United States do not meet CDC criteria whereas 60% are "very inactive." When the risk of heart disease among active people is compared to very inactive people, the risk in the inactive segment was twice that of individuals in the active population. To put this in perspective, as the authors of this study did, this means that individuals who choose to be inactive accept the same increased risk of heart disease as individuals who smoke a pack of cigarettes a day! Unfortunately, 15% of the adult population in the United States still smoke a pack of cigarettes a day whereas 60–80% of adults are either not adequately active or completely inactive. Thus, inactivity carries the same risk as smoking a pack of cigarettes per day and is between 4 and 5 times more prevalent! We have an enormous opportunity to engage the American public in ways of becoming more physically active to combat the adverse health effects of the epidemic of inactivity in the United States.

Despite the enormous amount of information available on the links between physical activity and health, the medical community has been slow to incorporate this information into the routine practice of medicine. Studies have shown that less than 40% of physicians ever counsel people on physical activity. This is an unfortunate, wasted opportunity given that 70% of the individuals in the United States see their primary care physician at least once per year.

The evidence for both lifestyle medicine and physical activity is based on the enormous strength of the research literature in these areas and underscored by their incorporation into virtually every evidence-based clinical guideline addressing prevention and treatment of metabolic diseases. For example, the following guidelines and consensus statements of various prestigious medical organizations all provide significant emphasis on both lifestyle medicine principles and practices in general, as well as regular physical activity as a key component of the prevention and treatment of disease.

- JNC VIII Guidelines for Hypertension, Prevention and Treatment
- ACC/AHA Guidelines for the Prevention, Detection, Evaluation and Treatment of High Blood Pressure
- NCEP (ATP IV) Guidelines for Blood Cholesterol
- Institute of Medicine Guidelines for Obesity Treatment
- ACC/AHA Scientific Consensus Statement on the Treatment for Blood Cholesterol
- Guidelines from the American Diabetes Association for the Management of Diabetes
- Dietary Guidelines for Americans 2015-2020
- American Heart Association Nutrition Implementation Guidelines
- Guidelines from the American Academy of Pediatrics for the Prevention and Treatment of Childhood Obesity
- Guidelines from the American Academy of Pediatrics for the Treatment of Pediatric Blood Pressure
- Guidelines from the American Academy of Pediatrics for the Treatment of Lipids
- Guidelines from the American Heart Association and the American Academy of Pediatrics for the Prevention and Treatment of the Metabolic Syndrome
- American Heart Association Strategic Plan for 2020
- Joint Statement from the American Heart Association and American Cancer Society for the Prevention of Heart Disease and Cancer
- Presidential Advisory from the AHA and American Stroke Association on Optimal Brain Health
- AHA/ACC/TOS Guideline for the Management of Overweight and Obesity in Adults
- ACS/ADA/AHA Scientific Statement on Preventing Cancer, Cardiovascular Disease and Diabetes
- Physical Activity Guidelines Advisory Committee Report of 2018

Increasing physical activity in the population of the United States and other industrialized countries could carry enormous positive public-health implications. For example, consider the following known benefits of regular physical activity.

- Reduction of the risk of cardiovascular disease, which remains the leading killer of both men and women in the United States

- Reduction in the risk of type 2 diabetes, which is found in 10–12% of the population in the United States
- Reduction in the likelihood of prediabetes advancing to diabetes. (Estimates range from 36% to 38% of the adult population who have prediabetes)
- Reduction in the likelihood of weight gain and overweight or obesity
- Significant reduction in both systolic and diastolic blood pressure, which is the leading risk factor for cardiovascular disease and found in almost half of the population in the United States
- Reduction in the risk of osteoarthritis and assistance in its treatment
- Reduction in sedentary lifestyle, which has become a significant risk factor for multiple chronic diseases
- Reduction of the risk of multiple cancers
- Reduction in stress and likelihood of anxiety and depression

The power of physical activity as part of an overall program of positive lifestyle practices and habits has been shown in multiple, large randomized trials. For example, in the Diabetes Prevention Program, individuals with baseline glucose intolerance who increased physical activity and lost 5–7% of their body weight reduced their risk of developing diabetes by 58%. In the Look AHEAD trial, individuals with diabetes who exercised between 150 and 175 minutes of moderate physical activity per week and lost 7% of their body weight substantially lowered their risk of heart disease. Importantly, in both of these studies levels of physical activity and maintenance of weight loss were maintained in over four years of follow-up.

Connecting lifestyle medicine to physical activity gives me an opportunity to combine two areas where I am passionately committed. I had the honor of naming the field of lifestyle medicine in the academic literature with the publication of the first edition of my comprehensive textbook, *Lifestyle Medicine* (Blackwell Science, 1999). In this book I summarized the field of lifestyle medicine as the discipline of studying how daily habits and actions impact on short- and long-term health and quality of life. This textbook is now in its third edition, which came out in 2019. It is a massive 1,500-page textbook with over 200 contributors. I served as its Editor in Chief. I also am the Editor in Chief of the only academic journal in this area (the *American Journal of Lifestyle Medicine*; SAGE Publications). I have also been a lifelong exerciser, and my research team and I have published numerous articles and books in this area.

The field of lifestyle medicine has grown rapidly over the past two decades since the publication of my first textbook in this area. There is now an academic organization devoted entirely to lifestyle medicine, the American College of Lifestyle Medicine. In addition, the Council of the American Heart Association on which I sit changed its name from the "Nutrition, Physical Activity and Metabolic Council" to the "Council on Lifestyle and Cardiometabolic Health." The American Academy of Family Practice as well as the American College of Preventive Medicine now offer education tracks for individuals interested in adding lifestyle medicine as a key component of their medical practices.

There is no question that we need to find ways of engaging the American population in understanding the importance of what each person does on a daily basis. We basically have developed a medical system that is essentially disease- and sickness-oriented rather than lifestyle- and prevention-oriented. This has happened despite the fact that it is now estimated that over 80% of all illnesses have a significant lifestyle component.

The expense of a system that focuses on treating diseases rather than promoting a healthy lifestyle is obvious. We currently spend over 17% of the Gross National Product in the United States on what is basically sickness care. This is not a long-term solution and is rapidly becoming financially unsustainable.

Thus, lifestyle medicine is destined to play a significant role in helping to under-score the reality of how lifestyle habits and practices contribute to good health. Conversely, the absence of positive behaviors contributes in major ways to disease.

The current monograph focuses on physical activity for a variety of reasons. First, as already indicated, there is an enormous body of literature showing how physical activity plays critical roles in reducing virtually every form of disease and condition throughout the lifespan. Second, it is an area in which I am particularly interested as a lifelong enthusiast of physical activity and as a researcher in this area. In fact, my research laboratory performed some of the key research projects in the area of walk-ing and health. Our work has been credited with providing fundamental information to spur the modern American walking movement.

This current book focuses on how physical activity can make significant health contributions throughout the lifespan. The book starts with a general description of how physical activity impacts on health and why it is such a critical component of lifestyle medicine. The discussion then moves on to providing a description of key physical activity concepts. This is important to make sure that everyone fundamen-tally understands the key concepts related to physical activity. The book then moves forward to explore physical activity and the risks of various chronic diseases such as cardiovascular disease, cancer, diabetes and prediabctes, and the metabolic syn-drome. A whole chapter is devoted to the role of physical activity in the prevention of weight gain and in the treatment of obesity and another entire chapter is devoted to the role of physical activity in cognition and brain health.

The discussion then turns to the importance of physical activity in various popu-lations including the important information available for physical activity in wom-en's health, children, and youth, physical activity in older patients as well as those with chronic conditions.

The book continues with chapters on the important role that physicians play in promoting physical activity as well as some specific information gleaned from the 25 years that my research team has worked in the area of physical activity and health where I outline our approach to exercise prescription both in healthy individuals and special populations. There has been recent interest in the multiple adverse health consequences of sedentary behavior, so an entire chapter is devoted to this.

Finally, since behaviors such as physical activity do not take place in a vacuum, a discussion is included about the various factors that impact on the likelihood that individuals will engage in regular physical activity. Some of these are individual factors but there are also community factors as well as public health policies and built-in environment factors. In each of these areas, there is enormous evidence of the profound impact of physical activity on health along with ways to positively impact on physical activity.

This book represents the first book in a series for which I am proud to serve as Series Editor on various issues in lifestyle medicine. Other volumes in this series will include *Lifestyle Medicine: Cardiovascular Disease Prevention and Treatment, Lifestyle Medicine: Obesity Prevention and Treatment, Lifestyle Medicine: Behavior Change and Coaching,* and *Lifestyle Medicine: Plant Based Eating and Health.*

There will be further volumes in addition to these over the next few years. The attempt of these smaller volumes is to provide a point of entry for individuals who have a specific interest or want an in-depth exploration of a particular aspect of life-style medicine. I also hope to provide a point of entry for medical students and other students who are at the early stages in their careers and might find the price point of the major textbook that I edit in lifestyle medicine overwhelming.

In the final analysis, the habits and practices each of us engage in on a daily basis profoundly affect our health. By starting this series with the critically important area of physical activity, I hope to underscore the fact that simple changes in regular physical activity can exert enormous positive benefits. These are not only fitness benefits but also benefits in the reduction of risk in a variety of various diseases and conditions ranging from cardiovascular disease to cancer and diabetes. Increased physical activity also profoundly affects important areas such as cognition, mental health, and prevention of dementia.

There is no longer any serious doubt that we need to emphasize the multiple positive benefits of physical activity to the American public. I hope that books in the "Lifestyle Medicine" series will further educate and inspire health-care professionals and the public at large in making positive lifestyle decisions that will have a significant and positive impact on health. This is, in fact, the mandate that we have in American medicine and the reason why each of us chose to enter this sacred field.

James M. Rippe, MD
Boston, MA

Acknowledgments

Textbook writing and editing are collaborative efforts that involve the hard work and passion of numerous contributors. Many individuals over my 30-plus years as a physician have stimulated and influenced my thinking about the interaction between lifestyle and health, and the specific interactions between physical activity and good health, productivity, and enhanced quality of life.

Too many individuals fit into this category to acknowledge all by name; however, I would like to particularly thank a few individuals who have made substantial contributions to the current book.

First, my long-term Editorial Director, Beth Grady, who plays a critically important role in all of the major writing and editing projects that emerge from my research organization deserves special thanks. This book is one of over 53 books that Beth has managed, which have been generated through our organization. In addition to the current textbook, Beth provides editorial direction to two academic journals that I edit as well as my major Lifestyle Medicine textbook (*Lifestyle Medicine*, Rippe J (editor) CRC Press, 2019) and our major intensive care textbook (*Irwin and Rippe's Intensive Care Medicine*, 8th edition, Wolters Kluwer, 2018). Beth possesses not only superb editorial skills but also an exceptional work ethic and unfailing good humor to make all of these complex and difficult projects possible.

I would also like to express my appreciation to our office support staff including my Executive Assistant, Carol Moreau, who seamlessly coordinates my schedule and travel plans to free up the time necessary for such large writing and publishing projects. Our Editorial Office Assistant, Deb Adamonis, assists all of us in the multiple daily tasks required to expedite diverse projects in our office; our Chief Financial Officer, Connie Martell, makes sure that the financial processes are in place so that all our projects move forward smoothly. The research team at Rippe Lifestyle Institute has always contributed enormous insights to clarify my thinking about a number of aspects of lifestyle medicine while our Director of Marketing and Client Services, Amy Continelli, coordinates daily interactions with multiple research sponsors.

I would also like to thank the outstanding editorial team at Taylor & Francis Group/CRC Press. Randy Brehm, Senior Editor, has been an early key supporter of our textbooks and Julia Tanner coordinated all aspects of the publication process and provided important day-to-day leadership and invaluable assistance on multiple issues related to manuscripts. Also Marsha Hecht at Taylor & Francis Group/CRC Press who managed every step of the production process with expertise, patience and knowledge. Finally, Rajiv Kumar at Cenveo Publisher Services who managed the editing design and typesetting of the book with great skill.

Finally, I am grateful to my family including my loving wife Stephanie Hart Rippe and our four beautiful daughters, Hart, Jaelin, Devon, and Jamie, who continue to love and support me through the arduous process of many major textbooks and journals and the other diverse professional responsibilities that I juggle, along with my family life.

If there are errors or omissions in *Increasing Physical Activity: A Practical Guide* the responsibility is mine. If there is credit due for this project, it belongs to the numerous people who have made substantial contributions to my knowledge and performance along the way.

James M. Rippe, M.D.
Boston, MA

Author Biography

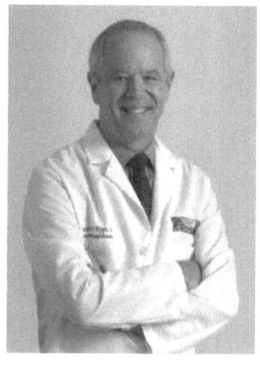

Dr James M. Rippe is a graduate of Harvard College and Harvard Medical School with postgraduate training at Massachusetts General Hospital. He is currently the Founder and Director of the Rippe Lifestyle Institute and Professor of Medicine at the University of Massachusetts Medical School.

Over the past 25 years Dr Rippe has established and run the largest research organization in the world exploring how daily habits and actions impact short- and long-term health and quality of life. This organization, Rippe Lifestyle Institute (RLI), has published hundreds of papers that form the scientific basis for the fields of lifestyle medicine and high-performance health. RLI also conducts numerous studies every year on physical activity, nutrition, and healthy weight management.

A lifelong and avid athlete, Dr Rippe maintains his personal fitness with a regular walk, jog, swimming, and weight training program. He holds a black belt in karate and is an avid wind surfer, skier, and tennis player. He lives outside of Boston with his wife Stephanie Hart—television news anchor—and their four children, Hart, Jaelin, Devon, and Jamie.

1 Lifestyle Medicine, Physical Activity, and Health

KEY POINTS

- Increased physical activity plays a variety of beneficial roles for individuals at all stages of their lives.
- Increased physical activity lowers the risk of various chronic diseases and also serves as an adjunct to their treatment.
- Recommendations to participate in 150 minutes of moderate or vigorous physical activity or more each week and strength training twice a week are guidelines that are shared by the Physical Activity Guidelines Advisory Council 2018, the American College of Sports Medicine, the American Heart Association, and other prestigious organizations.
- Physicians play a critically important role in urging people to make positive decisions in their lives concerning the level of physical activity.
- Currently, only 25% of individuals engage in regular levels of physical activity necessary to meet the guidelines from the Centers for Disease Control and Prevention and the American College of Sports Medicine.

1.1   INTRODUCTION

What each of us does in our daily lives profoundly impacts our short- and long-term health and quality of life. The study of these daily habits including proper nutrition, regular physical activity, weight management, and many other practices has now been lumped together under the umbrella term "lifestyle medicine." My research organization, Rippe Lifestyle Institute (RLI), coined this term in the academic literature with the publication of our first, major multi-authored textbook in this area *Lifestyle Medicine* (Blackwell Science, 1999) (1). Since that time, the field has continued to grow and prosper.

Amongst the many important things that each of us can do in our daily lives, there is no single lifestyle habit or practice that is more powerfully associated with improved short- and long- term health and quality of life than regular physical activity.

There is an enormous and compelling literature generated over the past two decades that documents that regular physical activity profoundly affects both the likelihood of developing chronic disease and also quality of life (2). In addition, regular physical activity has been shown in numerous studies to play a powerful role in not only the reduction of risk of various chronic diseases, but also as an adjunct to their treatment.

For all of these reasons, regular physical activity is a cornerstone in the prevention and treatment of chronic diseases and acknowledged as such by guidelines from numerous organizations ranging from the American Heart Association (AHA) (3), American Diabetes Association (ADA) (4), American Academy of Pediatrics (AAP), and many others (5–15). A partial list of the organizations that have recommended regular physical activity as a key component of positive health is found in Table 1.1 (6).

Regular physical activity is also a cornerstone of the recommendations for Healthy People 2020 (7) and a key factor in the framework that has been established for Healthy People 2030 (8). Recently, the Physical Activity Guidelines Advisory Committee Scientific Report for Americans (2018) was released providing an enormous compendium of new evidence about the multiple benefits of regular physical activity. Organizations such as the American College of Sports Medicine (ACSM) (9), the American College of Lifestyle Medicine (ACLM) (10), and the AHA (11) have also included recommendations for regular physical activity as a key component of preserving health and improving quality of life.

Despite the enormous information available till now concerning the relationship between regular physical activity and health, the medical community has been slow to specifically embrace this concept as a component of routine healthcare. It has

---

TABLE 1.1
Sampling of Guidelines That Incorporate Lifestyle Recommendations for the Treatment or Prevention of Chronic Disease

- ACC/AHA Guidelines for the Prevention, Detection, Evaluation, and Management of High Blood Pressure in Adults
- Institute of Medicine Guidelines for Obesity Management
- Dietary Guidelines for Americans 2015–2020
- Guidelines from the American Academy of Pediatrics for the Prevention and Treatment of Childhood Obesity
- Guidelines from the American Academy of Pediatrics for Heart Disease Risk Factor Reduction in Children
- American Heart Association Strategic Plan for 2020
- Preventing Cancer, Cardiovascular Disease, and Diabetes: A Common Agenda for the American Cancer Society, the American Diabetes Association, and the American Heart Association
- Defining Optimal Brain Health in Adults: A Presidential Advisory from the American Heart Association/American Stroke Association
- 2013 AHA/ACC/TOS Guideline for the Management of Overweight and Obesity in Adults
- 2018 Physical Activity Advisory Committee Scientific Report

Source: James M. Rippe, MD

been estimated that less than 40% of physicians regularly counsel their patients on the importance of increasing physical activity (12). Since over 70% of individuals see their primary care physicians at least once per year, this is clearly a wasted opportunity!

The American public has also been slow to embrace the habit of daily, regular physical activity. It is estimated that less than 25% of adults in the United States achieve the recommended levels of physical activity, including 30 minutes of moderate physical activity on most, if not all, days and two sessions of musculoskeletal strength training on a weekly basis (13). Clearly, we have a long way to go.

The purpose of this book is to summarize key elements of how physical activity plays an important role in health and quality of life. The intended audience for this book is physicians and other healthcare workers in the hope that these professionals will lead the charge to help individuals understand the power of their daily lifestyle habits and actions, in general, and the key role that regular physical activity specifically can play in enhancing health and lowering the risk of chronic disease.

1.2   THE RELATIONSHIP BETWEEN MODERATE TO VIGOROUS PHYSICAL ACTIVITY AND THE RISK OF DEVELOPING CHRONIC DISEASES

Enormous data are now available across a wide spectrum of chronic diseases to show that physically active individuals decrease their risk of these conditions compared to inactive individuals (2). Some of these benefits can even come after an acute bout of physical activity, while others require a consistent increase in physical activity throughout the lifespan. These conditions include reduction in the risk of cardiovascular disease (CVD), cancer, diabetes, dementia, and the risk of falling and injury, particularly in older individuals (2).

Multiple benefits also accrue to children as young as 3 years old, all the way up through adolescence. A summary of the activity-related health benefits documented in the 2018 Physical Activity Guidelines Advisory Committee Report is given in Table 1.2.

There is also a strong relationship between increased physical activity and quality of life. Individuals who are physically active, in general, feel better and sleep better. In addition, regular physical activity reduces the risk of anxiety and stress as well as depression (2). All of these improvements result in higher quality of life for individuals who participate in regular physical activity.

1.3   PHYSICAL ACTIVITY AND CHRONIC DISEASES

1.3.1   Cardiovascular Disease

Regular physical activity lowers the risk of CVD as well as all-cause mortality (14). In fact, even very small amounts of regular physical activity can result in significant lowering of the risk of both CVD and all-cause mortality. As shown

TABLE 1.2

Physical Activity-Related Health Benefits for the General Population and Selected Populations Documented by the 2018 Physical Activity Guidelines Advisory Committee

Children	
3 to <6 years of age	**Improved bone health and weight status**
6–17 years of age	**Improved cognitive function (ages 6–13 years)**
	Improved cardiorespiratory and muscular fitness
	Improved bone health
	Improved cardiovascular risk factor status
	Improved weight status or adiposity
	Fewer symptoms of depression
Adults, All Ages	
All-cause mortality	Lower risk
Cardiometabolic conditions	Lower cardiovascular incidence and mortality (including heart disease and stroke)
	Lower incidence of hypertension
	Lower incidence of type 2 diabetes
Cancer	Lower incidence of **bladder**, breast, colon, **endometrium, esophagus, kidney, stomach, and lung cancers**
Brain health	**Reduce risk of dementia**
	Improved cognitive function
	Improved cognitive function following bouts of aerobic activity
	Improved quality of life
	Improved sleep
	Reduced feelings of anxiety and depression in healthy people and in people with existing clinical syndromes
	Reduce incidences of depression
Weight status	**Reduced risk of excessive weight gain**
	Weight loss and the prevention of weight regain following initial weight loss when a sufficient dose of moderate-to-vigorous physical activity is attained
	An additive effect on weight loss when combined with moderate dietary restriction
Older Adults	
Falls	Reduce incidence of falls
	Reduce incidence of fall-related injuries
Physical function	**Improved physical function in older adults with and without frailty**
Women Who Are Pregnant or Postpartum	
During pregnancy	**Reduced risk of excessive weight gain**
	Reduced risk of gestational diabetes
	No risk to fetus from moderate-intensity physical activity
During postpartum	**Reduced risk of postpartum depression**

(*Continued*)

TABLE 1.2 (*Continued*)

Physical Activity-Related Health Benefits for the General Population and Selected Populations Documented by the 2018 Physical Activity Guidelines Advisory Committee

Individuals with Preexisting Medical Conditions	
Breast cancer	**Reduced risk of all-cause and breast cancer mortality**
Colorectal caner	**Reduced risk of all-cause and colorectal cancer mortality**
Prostate cancer	**Reduced risk of prostate cancer mortality**
Osteoarthritis	**Decreased pain**
	Improved function and quality of life
Hypertension	**Reduced risk of progression of cardiovascular disease**
	Reduced risk of increased blood pressure over time
Type 2 diabetes	**Reduced risk of cardiovascular mortality**
	Reduced progression of disease indicators: hemoglobin A1c, blood pressure, blood lipids, and body mass index
Multiple sclerosis	**Improved walking**
	Improved physical fitness
Dementia	**Improved cognition**
Some conditions with impaired executive function (attention deficit hyperactivity disorder, schizophrenia, multiple sclerosis, Parkinson's disease, and stroke)	**Improved cognition**

Benefits in **bold** font are those added in 2018; benefits in normal font are those noted in the 2008 Scientific Report. Only outcomes with strong or moderate evidence of effect are included in the table.

Source: 2018 Physical Activity Guidelines Advisory Committee Scientific Report. Washington, DC. Part D: Integrating the Evidence. D5-6.

in Figure 1.1, there is no lower threshold for the benefit of increased physical activity with regard to reduction of risk of all-cause mortality.

Individuals who engage in moderate or vigorous physical activity as low as 30 minutes per week can achieve significant benefits. Additional benefits accrue in individuals who achieve physical activity of 150–300 minutes of moderate or vigorous physical activity as shown in Figure 1.1.

Despite the known benefits of physical activity for reduction in the risk of coronary heart disease (CHD), substantially fewer than half of adults meet even the minimum recommendation for regular aerobic physical activity. Young people are even less likely to meet recommended standards with fewer than 20% of adolescents performing the recommended 60 minutes or more of daily physical activity (13).

Compared with those who are very physically active the risk of CHD in sedentary individuals is 150–240% higher. Unfortunately, only about 25% of Americans engage in the minimum standards recommended by the Centers for Disease Control and Prevention and the Physical Activity Guidelines for Americans 2018 guidance of at least 150 minutes per week of moderate intensity aerobic activity or at least

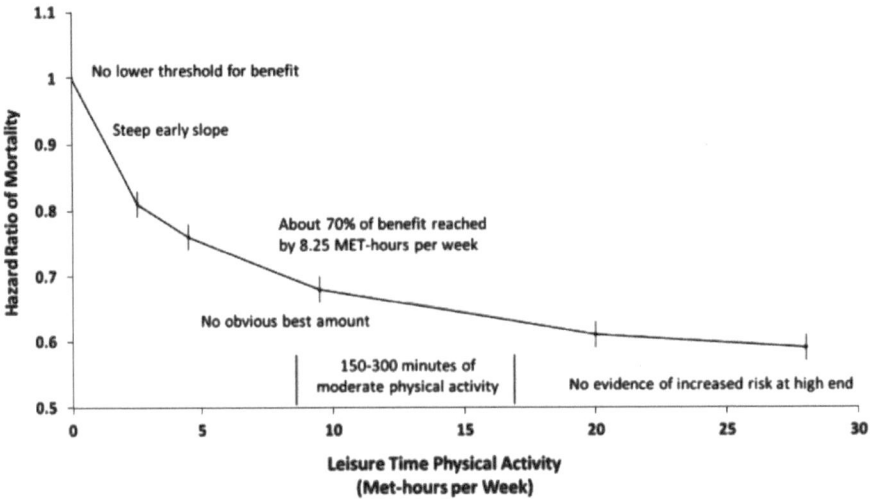

FIGURE 1.1 Relationships of moderate-to-vigorous physical activity to all-cause mortality, with highlighted characteristics common to studies of this type. (From the 2018 Physical Activity Guidelines Advisory Committee Scientific Report. Adapted from Moore SC, et al. Leisure time physical activity of moderate to vigorous intensity and mortality. A large pooled cohort study analysis. PloS Med. 2012:9 e1001335.)

75 minutes of vigorous exercise and muscle strengthening activities at least two days per week (2, 16). Regular physical activity also lowers the risk of adult weight gain and helps to control high blood pressure, while reducing the risk of developing hypertension in the first place. Increasing amounts of physical activity also lower the risk of stroke and heart failure with a dose dependent relationship.

Despite, these known benefits, physicians have not adequately emphasized the role of regular physical activity in reducing the risk of heart disease. In one survey of 175 primary care physicians, only 12% were aware of the recommendations from the ACSM, which mirror those of the PAGA 2018 (17). Detailed information about the relationship between physical activity and CVD risk factors may be found in Chapter 3.

1.3.2 PHYSICAL ACTIVITY AND DIABETES, PREDIABETES AND THE METABOLIC SYNDROME

Lifestyle modalities, including physical activity, are the cornerstone of diabetes care. People with diabetes should be encouraged to perform aerobic and resistance training regularly (3). According to guidelines from the American Diabetes Association, aerobic activity sessions should ideally be at least 10 minutes, with the goal of 30 minutes, per day or more on most days of the week.

In addition, individuals with diabetes should be encouraged to reduce the time spent on sedentary activities such as working on a computer, watching TV, or other periods of sitting or lying down (except sleep), or by breaking up sedentary activities by briefly standing, walking, or performing light physical activity.

The ADA Consensus Report on Physical Activity and Diabetes recommends that prior to starting an exercise program (18), medical providers should perform a careful history to assess cardiovascular risk factors and customize exercise regimens to individual needs. The role of regular physical activity in diabetes prevention and care is spelled out both in the guidelines from the American Diabetes Association as well as the PAGA 2018.

Multiple lifestyle interventions also play critically important roles in preventing prediabetes from turning into diabetes. Physical activity is a key component of these interventions. The Diabetes Prevention Program (DPP) demonstrated that intensive lifestyle intervention in individuals with prediabetes could reduce the incidence of type 2 diabetes (T2DM) by 58% over 3 years (19). The Da Qing Study (20) and Finnish Diabetes Prevention Study (21) showed similar reductions in the likelihood of prediabetes turning to diabetes. In the DPP, 150 minutes of physical activity, in addition to healthy weight and a 7% weight loss, was recommended to individuals with prediabetes.

1.3.3 THE METABOLIC SYNDROME

The metabolic syndrome is a cluster of metabolic abnormalities that significantly increase the risk of CVD (22). Increased physical activity represents a core intervention for individuals with the metabolic syndrome including proper nutrition (following either a DASH or Mediterranean or comparable diet) and regular physical activity of 30 minutes or more on most, if not all, days. A detailed summary of the role of physical activity and diabetes, prediabetes, and the metabolic syndrome is found in Chapter 5.

1.4 PHYSICAL ACTIVITY AND WOMEN'S HEALTH, INCLUDING PREGNANCY

Regular physical activity is an important lifestyle behavior for women throughout their lifespan (23). The guidelines from the AHA, the ACSM, and the PAGA 2018 all recommend 30 minutes of moderate intensity aerobic activity on most days of the week or 75 minutes per week of vigorous intensity physical activity.

Women who engage in walking 1.5 miles per week or more reduced their risk of heart disease by over 30% in the Women's Health Trial (24). Other studies including the National Institute of Health (NIH) AARP Diet and Health Study showed similar reductions in risk of heart disease for women who engaged in 20 minutes or more three times per week of moderate intensity physical activity (25). Regular physical activity has also been shown to lower the risk of excessive weight gain during pregnancy and reducing the risk of gestational diabetes (26). A more detailed exploration of the relationship between regular physical activity and women's health may be found in Chapter 12.

1.5 PHYSICAL ACTIVITY, WEIGHT GAIN, AND OBESITY

It is currently estimated that 78 million individuals in the United States are obese (27). This represents 36% of the population. More than 70% of the adults in the United States are either overweight (BMI $\geq$25 kg/m^2), obese (BMI $\geq$30 kg/m^2), or severely obese (BMI $\geq$35 kg/m^2).

Regular physical activity can reduce the risk of both weight gain and is also vitally important in maintaining weight loss (28). There is also an additive effect on weight loss when combining physical activity with moderate dietary restriction (29). In addition, regular physical activity in individuals who are overweight or obese conveys multiple benefits in reducing risk of various chronic diseases whether or not weight loss is achieved. More detail about the relationship between regular physical activity and lowering the risk of weight gain and the effects in obesity may be found in Chapter 8.

1.6 PHYSICAL ACTIVITY AND ITS RELATIONSHIP TO BRAIN HEALTH AND COGNITION

An important relationship exists between regular physical activity and various aspects of cognition and brain health (30). This aspect of physical activity is often underestimated by both physicians and patients.

Regular physical activity has been demonstrated to improve cognitive function and lower the risk of all forms of dementia, including Alzheimer's disease (30). In addition, regular physical activity has been demonstrated to reduce feelings of anxiety and depression in healthy people and also lower these factors in individuals with existing clinical affective syndromes, such as reducing the risk of depression.

The PAGA 2018 (2) and the Presidential Advisory from the AHA and the American Stroke Association (ASA) recommend regular physical activity as a key modality for improving brain health and function (30). In fact, the AHA/ASA Presidential Advisory include physical activity as one of the key recommendation in their statement on "Optimizing Brain Health."

The relationship between regular physical activity and brain health is important throughout the lifespan, but particularly important as the population in the United States and other industrialized countries continues to age and the prevalence of cognitive decline and dementia increases.

1.7 PHYSICAL ACTIVITY IN YOUTH

Regular physical activity conveys multiple benefits for children. The 2008 PAGA (31) recommendations for the amount of physical activity in youth were confined mostly to children between the ages of 6 and 17, since inadequate data were available for children between the ages of 3 and 6.

In the PAGA 2018 (2) the recommendations for increased physical activity were extended to include both children between the ages of 3 and 6 and also children and adolescents between the ages of 6 and 17. In the age group of 3–6 years, regular physical activity has been demonstrated to yield improved bone health and weight status. In children between the ages of 6 and 17, regular physical activity has been shown to improve not only bone health and weight status but also cognitive function and cardiorespiratory and muscular fitness, while lowering risk of CVD and reducing symptoms of depression. A more detailed exploration of the linkage between physical activity and children is in Chapter 14.

1.8 PHYSICAL ACTIVITY AND OLDER ADULTS

In 2016, individuals over the age of 65 comprised about 13% of the United States population (32). The numbers are projected to reach 72.1 million (19%) of the total population by the Year 2030. Moreover, people over the age of 85 are projected to rise to 14.6 million by Year 2040.

Increased physical activity plays a number of important roles in older individuals. Individuals in this age group are particularly susceptible to cognitive decline and dementia, the risks of both of which have been demonstrated to be lower in individuals who are physically active. Moreover, falls and injuries are the leading cause of hospitalization and disability in this age group. Regular physical activity has been demonstrated to result in decreased incidence of falls and fall related injuries. Regular physical activity also delays age related declines in aerobic conditioning. Muscle strengthening and physical activity all are important, particularly for older individuals where loss of strength and lean muscle are often present. The relationship between physical activity and the older population is discussed in detail in Chapter 16

1.9 PHYSICAL ACTIVITY IN INDIVIDUALS WITH CHRONIC CONDITIONS

Regular physical activity has been associated with reduced risk of a variety of chronic conditions including a variety of cancers (e.g., breast cancer, colorectal cancer, prostate cancer), as well as decreased pain and improved function and improved quality of life in individuals with osteoarthritis (33). In addition, regular physical activity results in reduced risk of progression of CVD and helps lower risk of elevated blood pressure as well as serving as an important adjunct in treatment of blood pressure. Increased physical activity has been demonstrated to lower the risk of cardiovascular mortality and progression of disease indicators in individuals with T2DM including elevated hemoglobin A1c, elevated blood pressure, blood lipids, and BMI. In addition, regular physical activity has been shown to lower the risk of dementia and improve cognition in a variety of other neurologic problems. The role of increased physical activity in individuals with chronic conditions is discussed in more detail in Chapter 16.

1.10 OVERCOMING SEDENTRY BEHAVIOR

Increased scientific interest has been focused in the past two decades on overcoming sedentary behavior. Recent data from the U.S. National Health and Nutrition Examination Survey indicate that children and adults spend approximately 7.7 hours per day (55% of waking time) being sedentary (34). Sedentary behavior has been associated with increased risk of heart disease, diabetes, obesity, and the metabolic syndrome. Increased physical activity has been shown to lower the risks of sedentary behavior (35). In particular, the highest risk of CVD occurs in individuals who are the least active and get the least amount of physical activity. Higher levels of regular physical activity can largely ameliorate the health risks of sedentary behavior. The issue of sedentary behavior and the value of overcoming this with regular physical activity are discussed in detail in Chapter 16.

1.11   THE ROLE OF PHYSICANS IN PROMOTING INCREASED PHYSICAL ACTIVITY

Physician counseling has been shown to play an important role in multiple components of positive lifestyle behavior, including physical activity. Unfortunately, less than 40% of physicians routinely discuss physical activity with patients (12). Furthermore, a distinct minority (in some studies only 12%) of physicians are comfortable with the physical activity guidelines recommended by the ACSM and the PAGA 2008 and 2018 (13). Physician recommendation has been demonstrated in numerous studies to play a powerful role in helping patients take more positive steps in their lives. It has also been shown that physicians who are involved in regular physical activity in their own lives are much more likely to discuss these issues with their patients. These issues are discussed in more detail in Chapter 15.

1.12   EVALUATING PATIENTS FOR INCREASED PHYSICAL ACTIVITY AND PRESCRIBING INCREASED PHYSICAL ACTIVITY FOR HEALTHY INDIVIDUALS AND SPECIAL POPULATIONS

A variety of tools are available from the ACSM to assist physicians in evaluating individuals prior to recommending increased physical activity and providing exercise prescriptions both for healthy populations and those with chronic disease or other special populations (9). In many instances, a formal evaluation from a physician prior to advising patients to increase physical activity will not be necessary. However, there are some instances where evaluation from a physician who is knowledgeable about physical activity will be very helpful for both the safety and benefit of their patients. These issues are discussed in more detail in Chapters 3 and 5.

1.13   PUBLIC HEALTH CONSIDERATIONS

Various interventions can impact the likelihood of increasing physical activity (36). Some of these interventions take place on an individual level such as programs involving older adults, youth, and healthy adults. Some interventions are community based such as those that are school-based or community wide. Other impacts on the likelihood of engaging in physical activity may come from environmental or policy interventions such as infrastructure that emphasizes active transportation community design factors such as parks and open spaces that encourage hiking and other access to indoor and outdoor facilities may also promote increased physical activity. New technologies such as wearable activity monitors, telephone-assisted programs, web-based or internet-delivered programs, computer-tailored interventions, or mobile phone programs can also impact helping individuals to increase their level of physical activity. All of these factors will be considered in more detail in Chapter 20.

1.14   STEPS IN PROMOTING REGULAR PHYSICAL ACTIVITY

A number of behavioral strategies may be helpful in increasing the likelihood of regular physical activity and also reducing sedentary behavior. Since increasing regular physical activity typically involves a change in behavior, it is important that physicians and other healthcare professionals understand and use effective behavioral strategies upon which to base physical activity programs.

Adherence to positive lifestyle factors also remains a challenging area. Scientific statements from the AHA and the PAGA Scientific Report 2018 have emphasized the importance of implementing behavioral guidelines and multiple factors such as individual, familial, community, national, and other influences to make positive changes in the level of physical activity and other behavioral strategies (36). Furthermore, these same strategies can effectively be applied to reduce sedentary behavior. More detail on these considerations can be found in Chapters 4 and 20.

1.15 CONCLUSIONS

Increasing physical activity and other positive lifestyle measures play critically important roles in enhancing the health of individuals in the United States and other countries. Increased physical activity has been demonstrated to yield a variety of benefits including, reducing the risk of chronic diseases and/or often serving as an adjunct to their treatment. These include CVD, T2DM, weight gain and obesity, and brain health. Populations that can be benefited from increased physical activity include women at all stages of life including pregnancy, youth, older adults, and individuals with chronic conditions. Furthermore, the risk of sedentary behavior has become an important topic of research. Increased physical activity, of course, can play an element in reducing the risk of sedentary behavior.

Physicians and other healthcare professionals play an important role in promoting physical activity. This may come from counseling and encouraging individuals to increase their physical activity, but may also come from providing physical activity and fitness evaluations and exercise prescriptions. All of these considerations may be impacted by a variety of forces, including individual factors, family factors, community factors, and national and other policies. The role of increased physical activity is a very important issue for improving the health of individuals at all stages of their lives. Physicians and other healthcare professionals can play a vital role in encouraging their patients to become more physically active.

Many factors impact on the health of individuals. Physical activity will be the focus of this book. However, certainly healthy nutrition, weight management, not smoking, and other factors play prominent roles as well. All of these issues are components of the emerging field of lifestyle medicine, which is the discipline of exploring how daily habits and actions impact on short- and long-term health and quality of life. The interface between physical activity and other positive lifestyle factors will be emphasized throughout this book.

CLINICAL APPLICATIONS

- Physical activity plays an important role in both decreasing the risk of chronic diseases and also in serving as an adjunct to their treatment.
- Increased physical activity plays an important role in improving the quality of life for individuals.

- Physicians have not been as active as we should be in encouraging physical activity.
- Only one out of every five adults in the United States meets the guidelines from the Physical Activity Guidelines for Americans 2018 and ACSM for regular physical activity including engaging in 150 minutes or more moderate to vigorous physical activity per week and two sessions of musculoskeletal strength training per week.
- Counseling on physical activity and its benefits should be a routine part of every physician's encounter with patients.

REFERENCES

1. Rippe J. Lifestyle Medicine. Blackwell Science, Inc. (London), 1999.
2. 2018 Physical Activity Guidelines Advisory Committee. 2018 Physical Activity Guidelines Advisory Committee Scientific Report. Washington, DC: U.S. Department of Health and Human Services, 2018.
3. Eckel RH, Jakicic JM, Ard JD, deJesus JM, et al. 2013 AHA/ACC guideline on lifestyle management to reduce cardiovascular risk: A report of the American College of Cardiology/American heart association task force on practice guidelines. Circulation. 2014;129:S76–S99.
4. American Diabetes Association. Lifestyle management: Standards of Medical Care in Diabetes 2019. Diabetes Care 2019;42(Suppl. 1):S46–S60.
5. Andersen LB, Murray RG. Cardiovascular risk and physical activity in children. Lifestyle Medicine (3rd edition). CRC Press (Boca Raton), 2019.
6. Rippe JM. From the editor: The lifestyle movement continues to grow and thrive. Am J Lifestyle Med. 5:288–290, 2014.
7. Healthy People 2020 [Internet]. Washington, DC: U.S. Department of Health and Human Services, Office of Disease Prevention and Health Promotion. https://www.healthypeople.gov/ [Accessed January 6, 2020].
8. Healthy People 2030 [Internet]. Washington, DC: U.S. Department of Health and Human Services, Office of Disease Prevention and Health Promotion. Development of the National Health Promotion and Disease Prevention Objectives for 2030. https://www.healthypeople.gov/2020/About-Healthy-People/Development-Healthy-People-2030 [Accessed January 6, 2020].
9. American College Sports Medicine website: https://www.acsm.org/.
10. American College Lifestyle Medicine website: https://www.lifestylemedicine.org/
11. Lloyd-Jones D, Hong Y, Labarthe D, et al. Defining and setting national goals for cardiovascular health promotion and disease reduction: the American heart Association's strategic impact goal through 2020 and beyond. Circulation. 2010;121:586–613.
12. Kennedy M. What physicians need to know, do and say to promote physical activity. Lifestyle Medicine (3rd edition). CRC Press (Boca Raton), 2019.
13. Zoeller RF. Physical activity and fitness in the prevention of cardiovascular disease. Lifestyle Medicine (3rd edition). CRC Press (Boca Raton), 2019.
14. Rippe JM, Angelopoulos TJ. The rationale for intervention to reduce the risk of cardiovascular disease. In Rippe JM (ed): Lifestyle Medicine (3rd edition). CRC Press (Boca Raton), 2019.
15. Wilson P, Agostino R, Levy D, et al. Prediction of coronary heart disease using risk factor categories. Circulation. 1998;97:1837–1847.

16. Adult participation in aerobic and muscle-strengthening physical activities - United States, 2011. MMWR. 2013;62(17):326–330.
17. Blair S, Kohl H, Barlow C. Physical activity, physical fitness, and all-cause mortality in women: do women need to be active? J Am Coll Nutr. 1993;12:368–371.
18. American Diabetes Association. Lifestyle management: standards of medical care in Diabetes—2019. Diabetes Care. 2019;42(Supplement 1): S46–S60.
19. Reduction in the incidence type 2 diabetes with lifestyle intervention or metformin. N Engl J Med. 2002;346:393–403.
20. Pan X, Li G, Hu Y. Effects of diet and exercise in preventing NIDDM in people with impaired glucose tolerance: the Da Qing IGT and diabetes study. Diabetes Care 1997 Apr; 20(4): 537–544.
21. Lindstrom J, Louheranta A, Mannelin M, et al. The Finnish diabetes prevention study (DPS) lifestyle intervention and 3-year results on diet and physical activity. Diabetes Care 26:3230–3236, 2003.
22. Rippe J, Angelopoulos T. Preventing and managing obesity: The scope of the problem. In Rippe JM and Angelopoulos TA (eds). Obesity: Prevention and Treatment. CRC Press (Boca Raton, FL), 2012
23. Bassuk SS, Manson JE. Lifestyle and risk of cardiovascular disease and type 2 diabetes in women: a review of the epidemiologic evidence. Am J Lifestyle Med. 2008;2:191–213.
24. Manson J, Rich-Edwards J, Colditz A, et al. A prospective study of walking as compared with vigorous exercise in the prevention of coronary heart disease in women. N Engl J Med. 1999;341(9):650–658.
25. Lee I, Rexrode K, Cook N, et al. Physical activity and coronary heart disease in women: is "no pain, no gain" passé? JAMA. 2001;285(11):1447–1454.
26. American College Obstetricians and Gynecologists. https://www.acog.org/About-ACOG/ACOG-Departments/Deliveries-Before-39-Weeks/ACOG-Clinical-Guidelines [Accessed February 3, 2020].
27. Ng M, Fleming T, Robinson M, et al. Global, regional, and national prevalence of overweight and obesity in children and adults during 1980-2013: a systematic analysis for the global burden of disease study 2013. Lancet (London, England). 2014;384(9945):766–781.
28. Jakicic J, Rogers R, Collins K. Exercise management for the obese patient. Lifestyle Medicine (3rd edition). CRC Press (Boca Raton), 2019.
29. Wing R, Venditti E, Jakicic J, et al. Lifestyle intervention in overweight individuals with a family history of diabetes. Diabetes Care. 1998 Mar;21(3):350–359.
30. Gorelick P, Furie K, Iadecola C, et al. Defining optimal brain health in adults: a presidential advisory from the American heart association/American stroke association. Stroke.2017;48(10):e284–e303.
31. 2008 Physical Activity Guidelines Advisory Committee. 2018 Physical Activity Guidelines Advisory Committee Scientific Report. Washington, DC: U.S. Department of Health and Human Services, 2008.
32. 2018 Physical Activity Guidelines Advisory Committee. 2018 Physical Activity Guidelines Advisory Committee Scientific Report. Washington, DC: U.S. Department of Health and Human Services, 2018. Part F. Chapter 9. Older Adults: F9-1:F9-42
33. 2018 Physical Activity Guidelines Advisory Committee. 2018 Physical Activity Guidelines Advisory Committee Scientific Report. Washington, DC: U.S. Department of Health and Human Services, 2018. Part F. Chapter 10. Individuals With Chronic Conditions: F10-2:F10-101

34. Blodgett J, Theou O, Kirkland S, et al. The association between sedentary behaviour, moderate-vigorous physical activity and frailty in NHANES cohorts. Maturitas. 2015;80(2):187–191.
35. 2018 Physical Activity Guidelines Advisory Committee. 2018 Physical Activity Guidelines Advisory Committee Scientific Report. Washington, DC: U.S. Department of Health and Human Services, 2018. Part F. Chapter 2. Sedentary Behavior. F2-1.
36. 2018 Physical Activity Guidelines Advisory Committee. 2018 Physical Activity Guidelines Advisory Committee Scientific Report. Washington, DC: U.S. Department of Health and Human Services, 2018. Part F. Chapter 11. Promoting Physical Activity. F11-1.

2 Background and Key Physical Activity Concepts

KEY POINTS

- Increased physical activity has been demonstrated to yield multiple health benefits.
- This chapter provides core concepts that are important for every physician and health-care worker to understand when recommending increased physical activity.
- Though physical activity and physical fitness are inter-related, they are somewhat different terms and imply different ways of thinking about exercise or body movements.
- Physicians and other health-care workers should be knowledgeable about the terminologies and concepts related to physical activity so that they can more accurately counsel individual patients in these important areas.

2.1 INTRODUCTION

Over the past 30 years, the concept of physical activity and its role in improving health have developed rapidly and changed in meaningful ways (1).

From a historical perspective, initial work unfolded in the 1950s and 1960s in the area of exercise physiology largely to understand the heart disease epidemic. This included the inauguration of the landmark Framingham Study (2). The concern was that heart disease that was present only in 8–10% of the population in the 1920s had risen to almost 40% by 1960 (3).

There had been an historic belief in medicine that once a person had a heart attack, physical activity was contraindicated. The famous cardiologist, Paul Dudley White, however, who served as President Eisenhower's cardiologist, declared when the President had a heart attack in 1954 that he would be fine as long as he took up a regular program of walking. Dr. White's comments served as a wake-up call to physicians concerning the positive value of physical activity in not only the prevention, but also the treatment of heart disease.

Perhaps the next important milestone emerged in 1979 when the then Surgeon General Dr. Julius Richmond issued a Surgeon General's Report emphasizing the need for prevention of heart disease and other chronic diseases (4). His report followed a well-known report from the Canadian government in 1974 by the Canadian Minster of Health and Welfare Dr. Marc Lalonde, which was titled "A New Perspective on the Health of Canadians" and emphasized disease prevention and health promotion while calling attention to the importance of "lifestyle" practices including physical activity to reduce the risk of chronic diseases (5).

By the 1980s, a large body of scientific evidence had emerged and clearly demonstrated that regularly performing moderate to vigorous activities reduced the risk of heart disease and yielded other benefits.

As the field of physical activity and health continued to evolve, the Surgeon General's Report of 1996 (6) elaborated a similar message. In 2008 the first Physical Activity Guidelines for Americans (7) was published in an attempt to elevate the field of physical activity to the same scientific stature as the Dietary Guidelines for Americans (8).

Most recently, the Physical Activity Guidelines Advisory Committee Scientific Report 2018 (1) greatly expanded the findings of the preceding Physical Activity Report and listed a number of new areas and new conditions where regular physical activity had been shown to yield health benefits.

Thus, as the field of physical activity and health has matured, it was expanded to include not only exercise science and epidemiology, but also various aspects of behavioral and clinical science as well as city planning, political science, and many other disciplines (9).

While enormous advances have transpired in the area of physical activity and its role in health, the medical profession has not been as active as it should be in embracing this information and transferring it to patients. For example, less than 40% of physicians regularly counsel their patients on physical activity (10).

The purpose of this chapter is to provide a common understanding and terminology particularly for physicians and other health-care workers concerning terms that are central to the modern understanding of physical activity and health. The benefits of physical activity will also be put in the context of how other aspects of daily habits and actions impact on health. This area has been titled "Lifestyle Medicine," which will also be discussed in this chapter.

2.2 LIFESTYLE MEDICINE AND PHYSICAL ACTIVITY

An overwhelming body of scientific information has emerged over the past 20 years showing how daily habits and actions impact on short- and long-term health and quality of life. Since this information has emerged from a variety of disciplines, it may be difficult for physicians to develop a comprehensive knowledge of the evidence that has been developed. With this in mind, an academic field titled "Lifestyle Medicine" has evolved to help physicians and other health-care workers understand and employ this important body of information.

I am proud to have coined the term "lifestyle medicine" in the academic literature with the publication of my first comprehensive textbook in this area "Lifestyle Medicine" in 1999 (11). This book brought together the talents and expertise of over 150 scientists and researchers in diverse areas of physical activity, nutrition, weight management, behavioral medicine, and many other fields.

We defined lifestyle medicine in this 1999 textbook as "the discipline of studying how daily habits and practices impact both on prevention and treatment of disease often in conjunction with pharmaceutical or surgical therapy to provide an important adjunct to overall health." This basic definition has stood the test of time and is incorporated in subsequent editions of the lifestyle medicine textbook that I edit, the most recent one was published in 2019 (12). Though there have been a number of constructs concerning the concepts related to lifestyle medicine and many investigators have made important contributions to its components such as healthy nutrition, regular physical activity, weight management, and smoking cessation, it is clear that the field has now coalesced around the term "lifestyle medicine."

For example, The American Heart Association (AHA) changed the name of one of its councils from the "Council on Nutrition, Physical Activity and Metabolism" to the "Council on Lifestyle and Cardiometabolic Health" in 2013 (13). In addition, both the American College of Preventive Medicine and the American Academy of Family Practice have established working groups and educational tracks in the area of lifestyle medicine.

Importantly, a new professional organization for physicians and other healthcare workers has been formed and is called "The American College of Lifestyle Medicine" (ACLM) (14), which is devoted to providing a professional home and services for individuals who wish to emphasize lifestyle medicine in their practices. In addition, a peer reviewed, academic journal has been established, the *American Journal of Lifestyle Medicine*, to provide a forum for individuals interested in the exchange of evidence-based information in this growing field.

Though there are many components of lifestyle medicine, the area of physical activity remains critically important and for this reason this entire book is devoted to this area. Regular physical activity has been clearly demonstrated to reduce the risk of cardiovascular disease (CVD), type 2 diabetes (T2DM), the metabolic syndrome, obesity, and certain types of cancer (1). This important role for physical activity has been addressed, not only in the Physical Activity Guidelines for Americans 2018, but also in the guidelines from virtually every professional organization devoted to the study of metabolic disease (15). Thus, the field of lifestyle medicine has continued to grow. The pivotal concept of increased physical activity is a cornerstone of the study of how daily habits and actions impact on short- and long-term health and quality of life that is the essence of lifestyle medicine.

2.3 CORE TERMS

To explore the issue of physical activity and health, it is important to have a clear understanding of several core terms such as physical activity and exercise.

2.3.1 Physical Activity

Physical activity is any movement of the body produced by skeletal muscles that results in energy consumption. This term does not imply any specific aspect of the movement and is a broad concept encompassing a variety of types and intensities of movement. This term should be used for discussing a full range of activities all the way from sedentary behavior to light, moderate, or vigorous forms of physical movement.

2.3.2 Exercise

Exercise, in contrast to physical activity, is the type of activity that is planned, structured, repetitive, and designed to improve or maintain physical fitness, physical performance, or health. While this term has often been used to mean moderate or vigorous physical activity, it is more proper to use the term "exercise." Though physical activity and physical fitness are strongly inter-related, they are not exactly identical as will be discussed subsequently in this chapter.

2.4   TYPES OF PHYSICAL ACTIVITIES

Physical activities may be divided into the following types:

A. Aerobic physical activities—These include types of activities that are designed to be intense enough and performed long enough to improve an individual's cardiorespiratory fitness. Aerobic activities include such practices as walking, running, and basketball, which require repetitive use of large muscles. Aerobic physical activities include activities that are maintained by using only the oxygen-supported metabolic energy pathways and have typically come to mean activities expected to maintain or improve cardiorespiratory fitness.

B. Anaerobic physical activities—These types of physical activities involve high-intensity activities that exceed the normal capacity of the cardiovascular system to provide oxygen to muscle cells utilizing the usual oxygen that is delivered through the metabolic pathways. High-intensity interval training is a form of anaerobic physical activity. Anaerobic activity typically can only be maintained in bursts of 2–3 minutes.

C. Muscle strengthening activities—These are activities designed to improve muscular strength, endurance, or power. These can include everyday activities such as carrying heavy loads and shoveling snow but may also involve the use of exercise equipment such as machines, free weights, or elastic bands. Use of one's own body weight such as in push-ups or pull-ups is also considered muscular strengthening activity.

D. Bone strengthening activities—These are typically activities that create impact and muscle loading forces on bone. These types of activities put stress on the bones that adapt by modifying their structure or mass. This type of physical activity typically increases the resistance to bone fracture. Running, jumping, and dancing are good bone strengthening exercises, as are muscle strengthening exercises. It is important to understand that typically the bone building years occur in adolescence through young adulthood (i.e. the twenties). Of course, in addition to weight-bearing exercises, other factors such as appropriate amounts of calcium in the diet are also important for bone building.

E. Balance training—Movements that safely challenge postural control have been shown to improve balance and lower the risk of falling involve a variety of balance exercises that are described in more detail in subsequent chapters. These types of activities are particularly important for older individuals to decrease the likelihood of falls.

F. Flexibility training—Flexibility training may also be termed as "stretching." It is designed to lower the risk of joint injury and improve the range and ease of movement.

G. Yoga, Tai Chi, and Qigong—These activities typically involve muscle strengthening, balance training, and light intensity aerobic activity and flexibility. Some variations of these activities may also involve meditation and spirituality and, as a result, are sometimes called "mind/body" activities.

2.5 DOMAINS OF PHYSICAL ACTIVITY

A variety of constructs have been developed to classify physical activity. Of course, physical activity can happen at various times during the day, but one framework for domains of physical activity, which is outlined in the PAGA 2018 Scientific Report, involves the following four domains:

- Occupational physical activity (activity performed at work).
- Transportation physical activity (e.g. walking or bicycling to and from school or work or while shopping).
- Household physical activity (this is the activity done around one's home).
- Leisure time physical activity (sports, exercise, playing games, or going for a walk are examples of leisure time physical activities).

2.6 BODY POSITION

There has been recent interest in utilizing body position as one way of characterizing physical activity. Since a great deal of awake time is spent sitting, a good deal of research has focused on sitting. In addition, the definition of sedentary behavior used in the PAGA 2018 Scientific Report (1) is "any waking behavior characterized by an energy expenditure of less than or equal to 1.5 metabolic equivalents (METs), while in a sitting reclining or lying posture." This definition of sedentary behavior will be used throughout this book. (See also Chapter 15 for more details.)

2.7 ABSOLUTE VERSUS RELATIVE INTENSITY

The intensity of physical activity or exercise is an important concept that has been used extensively in exercise physiology. There are two broad classifications of intensity, either "absolute" intensity or "relative" intensity. Absolute intensity is the rate of energy expenditure required to perform any physical activity and is typically measured in METs. One MET is the rate of energy expenditure sitting at rest and is approximately 3.5 milliliters of oxygen/kilogram per minute. Absolute rates of energy expenditure are typically divided into four general classifications, as follows:

- Vigorous intensity activity—This requires 6.0 or greater METs. Examples include a very fast walking (4.5 miles/hour, running, swimming, or participating in aerobics classes). National data suggest that adults typically spend less than 1% of waking time in vigorous activity.
- Moderate intensity activity—This range is between 3.0 and less than 6.0 METs. Examples include brisk walking (3–4 miles/hour), raking a yard, or doing vigorous gardening.

- Light intensity activity—This is typically defined as 1.6 to less than 3.0 METs. A typical example would be slow or leisurely walking.
- Sedentary activity—This is physical activity requiring 1.0–1.5 METs. Typical examples include sitting and reading, screen time, television viewing, or similar activities. It has been estimated that adults in the United States spend more than 50% of their walking time in sedentary activities.

In contrast to absolute intensity, relative intensity represents a classification particularly appropriate for older individuals for whom a particular activity may be more difficult to perform than for younger individuals. Relative intensity denotes the difficulty an individual has in performing any given physical activity. Relative intensity is typically measured by the individual's perception of how difficult it is to perform a task or percentage of maximum heart rate. There are also scales of "perceived exertion" such as the Ten Point Scale of Perceived Exertion when performing a task. Moderate intensity physical activity is typically rated at 5 or 6 on the scale of 0–10, where "10" is the maximum exertion an individual is capable of. Vigorous activity is rated as somewhat higher at 7 or 8. Relative intensity is typically used to ensure that the level of physical activity is at the appropriate level for each individual and is particularly valuable for older individuals or individuals who have been previously sedentary.

2.8   DOSE, VOLUME, AND DOSE/RESPONSE

The dose of aerobic physical activity is typically noted by the acronym "FITT." This is widely used in exercise prescription and by most exercise physiologists. It is framed by the following concept:

- Frequency (either per day or per week).
- Intensity (energy expended during physical activity)
- Time (length of time for each session)
- Type (denotes the type of physical activity performed)

Volume denotes the amount of activity accumulated over a specified length of time. This could be per day, per week, or longer periods of time.

Dose/response is the relationship between the volume (dose) of physical activity and how the magnitude of the change in the health outcome or physiologic result (response). In most of the entities that are outlined in this book there is a definite dose/response relationship where increased amounts of physical activity result in more health benefits. An example of this is shown in Figure 2.1 (16).

Figure 2.1 shows that people who meet the guidelines of 150–300 minutes of moderate to vigorous physical activity on a weekly basis derive substantial benefits particularly compared to those individuals who are completely sedentary. As illustrated in Figure 2.1 there is also a significant benefit for people who engaged in even smaller amounts of physical activity. Thus, the take home message is that "some is

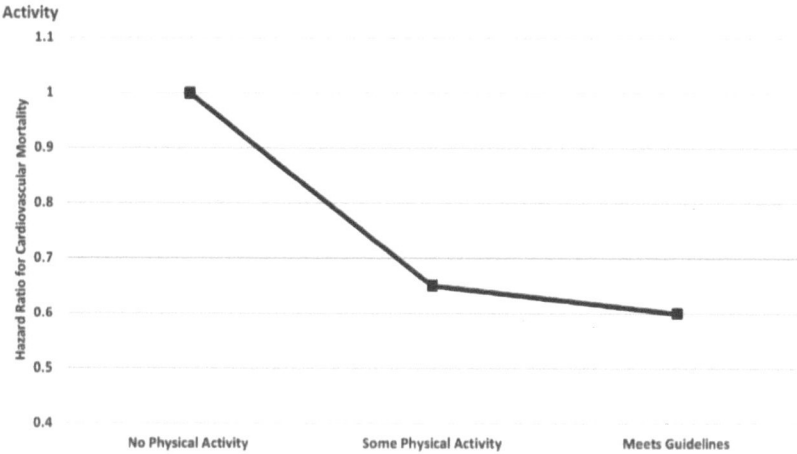

FIGURE 2.1 Risk of cardiovascular mortality among people with T2DM by dose of physical activity.

2018 Physical Activity Guidelines Advisory Committee. 2018 Physical Activity Committee Scientific Report. Washington, DC. US Department of Health and Human Services, 2018. Adapted from; Sadarangani K, Hamer M. Mindell J. et al. Physical Activity and Risk of all-cause and cardiovascular disease mortality in adults from Great Britain: Pooled analysis of 10 population-based cohorts. Diabetes Care. 2014;37:1016-1023.

better than none." This will be demonstrated in relation to multiple disease entities in subsequent chapters throughout this book.

2.9 MEASURING PHYSICAL ACTIVITY

It is important to make accurate measurements in order to make correlations between physical activity and health benefits. The ability to make these measurements has changed dramatically over the last three decades. The earliest estimates of physical activity came from occupational categories. This approach, however, was much more appropriate when the majority of workers had physically demanding jobs.

Estimates of occupational physical activity were subsequently replaced by questionnaires. Such questionnaires typically resulted from individuals reporting their own activity or from observers watching physical activity in others (e.g., in children). Most of the available questionnaires have categorized the amount of moderate or physical activity, although there are now some recently available questionnaires looking at sedentary behavior.

Devices used to measure physical movement have continued to evolve. Initially only pedometers were available that counted steps. Now devices that also have accelerometers that allow measurement of bodily movements are available. These more technologically advanced devices have led to the ability to use phone apps and components of wearable devices to make reasonably accurate estimates of the amount of physical activity individuals indulge in. It is anticipated that these devices will continue to become more widely used and precise. These devices can also measure steps and are typically paired with global positioning systems that provide estimates of speed and distance. Some of these devices also include heart rate monitors that allow estimates of relative and absolute energy expenditures.

2.10   MONITORING PHYSICAL ACTIVITY

Monitoring the relationship between physical activity and various health outcomes is important in order to make public health recommendations. This may involve not only measuring an individual's response to physical activity but also assessing other aspects of physical activity such as public policies and environments.

The ability to estimate levels of physical activity is very important to understand the proportions of individuals that perform different amounts of physical activity, as demonstrated in Figure 2.2.

As depicted in Figure 2.2, the majority of individuals in the United States are either inactive or insufficiently active. This figure shows how much opportunity exists for helping people understand the benefits of increased physical activity.

It has also been demonstrated that men are slightly more likely to obtain the recommended range of moderate to vigorous physical activity than women (55% compared to 45%) (17). High school boys are also substantially more likely to meet recommended aerobic target than high school aged girls (37% versus 17%). This disparity suggests that education starting at the high school level about the benefits of physical activity is very important, particularly for girls.

2.11   PHYSICAL FITNESS VERSUS PHYSICAL ACTIVITY

Though there is a correlation between physical fitness and physical activity, these terms define slightly different concepts. Physical fitness is a physiologic attribute assessing a person's ability to perform muscle powered work. It is defined by the American College of Sports Medicine (ACSM) as "the ability to deliver and utilize oxygen during sustained activity"; physical fitness is typically quantified as a percentage of maximum oxygen uptake (VO_{2max}). In contrast, physical activity is typically assessed by retrospective self-reported data (e.g., physical activity questionnaires).

The categorization of physical activity (i.e., low, moderate, or high) varies from study to study. ACSM defines moderate physical activity as any activity requiring 50–70% of VO_{2max} or 50–70% maximum heart rate (18). Vigorous physical activity is anything greater than 70% of VO_{2max} or 70% maximum heart rate. Walking or brisk walking is generally recommended as the type of exercise that meets the criteria for moderate physical activity. Running or fast swimming is typically considered vigorous physical activity. The precise definition of moderate physical activity, however, varies depending on the baseline fitness and background of individuals. For example, healthy, athletic individuals may find that this level of walking does not even qualify as moderate intensity, whereas elderly or very sedentary individuals may find this to be a "vigorous" activity.

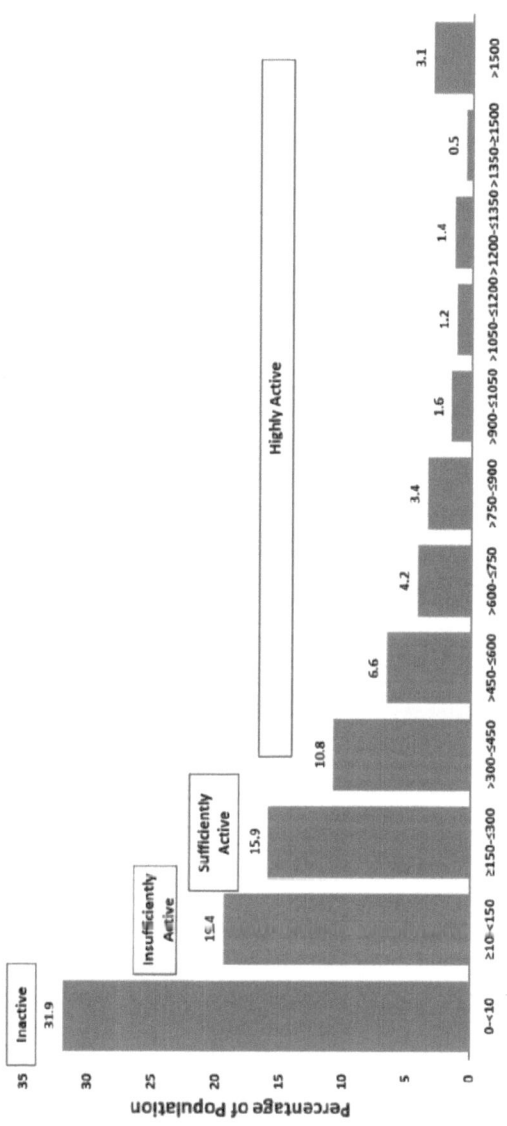

FIGURE 2.2 Distribution of self-reported volume of moderate-to vigorous physical activity, 150 minutes per week increments, US adults, 2015. 2018 Physical Activity Guidelines Advisory Committee. 2018 Physical Activity Guidelines Advisory Committee Scientific Report. Washington, DC: U.S. Department of Health and Human Services, 2018. Adapted from the data found in the National Health Interview Survey, 2015.

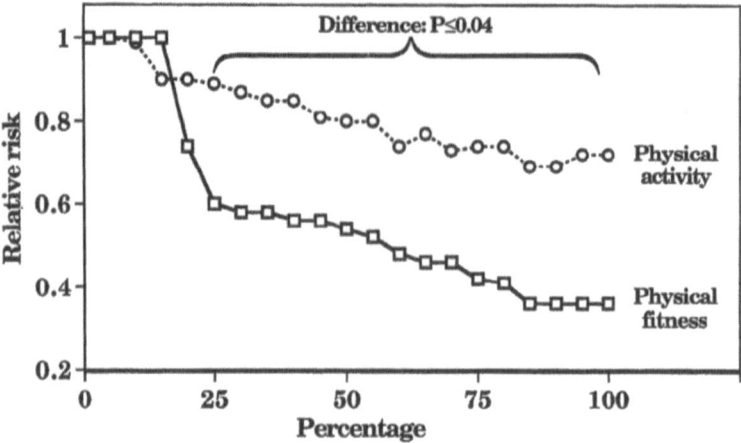

FIGURE 2.3   The relationship of physical fitness and physical activity to risk of heart disease.

Surprisingly, physical fitness has been only modestly correlated with physical activity. This is demonstrated in Figure 2.3, which shows that the relative risk of heart disease in individuals when measuring either physical activity or physical fitness varies considerably (19).

2.12   COMPONENTS OF PHYSICAL FITNESS

As defined by the ACSM and PAGA 2018 Scientific Report, there are five major components of physical fitness including the following:

- Cardiorespiratory endurance
- Musculoskeletal fitness
- Flexibility
- Balance
- Speed

It is important to emphasize that the scientific evidence shows that both physical activity and physical fitness provide important health benefits. As already indicated in Figure 2.1, some data suggest that physical fitness may be a more powerful indicator of reduction of risk of chronic disease than physical activity. Nonetheless, for most individuals the key issue is to increase levels of physical activity. This will be emphasized throughout this book.

2.13   PHYSICAL ACTIVITY ACROSS THE LIFESPAN

The capacity to perform physical activity as well as preferences and needs vary considerably across the lifespan. From a public health perspective, this means that guidelines need to be different for different age groups.

In current practice, the population is typically divided into three primary age groups: youth, adults, and older adults. The break between youth and adults usually denotes the transition from secondary school to either higher education or full-time work whereas the break between adults and older adults generally centers on retirement.

These breaks also typically represent factors that influence physical activity participation and, therefore, are important to take into consideration when developing programs to promote physical activity. The differences between capacity and preferences for these three age groups are handled in individual chapters on Youth, Adults, and Older Adults.

2.14 IDEAL CARDIOVASCULAR HEALTH

Organizations such as the AHA have become more actively involved in recognizing the importance of lifestyle issues and health; a few new terms have arisen that are important to understand. One of these is "Ideal" cardiovascular health. As defined in the AHA Strategic Plan for 2020 (20), this concept involves a variety of factors including physical activity, proper nutrition, no cigarette smoking, and healthy weight. In addition, a number of more medically related factors are incorporated into "ideal" cardiovascular health such as fasting blood glucose less than 100 mg/dL, untreated blood pressure of less than 130/80 mm/Hg, and untreated cholesterol less than 200 mg/dL. Though multiple factors play roles in "ideal" cardiovascular health, physical activity is central to this concept.

2.15 PRIMORDIAL PREVENTION

Primordial prevention is another concept that the AHA incorporated into their 2020 Strategic Plan. Primordial prevention extends the concept of risk factor reduction to eliminating risk factors in the first place rather than simply trying to reduce them. This concept shows that organizations such as the AHA are adopting an ever-more aggressive approach to helping people early in their lives lower their risk of heart disease. Increased physical activity plays a critically important role in the concept of primordial prevention.

2.16 OPTIMAL BRAIN HEALTH

Lifestyle factors including physical activity also play a very important role in brain health. The AHA and the American Stroke Association (ASA) emphasized this fact when they jointly issued a Presidential Advisory defining "Optimal Brain Health" in adults (21). This Presidential Advisory recognizes the strong relationship between cardiovascular risk factors and brain health risk factors.

Optimal brain health includes ways of maximizing cognitive function throughout a lifespan and lowering the risk of dementia. The AHA/ASA Presidential Advisory identified seven components that contribute to optimal brain health that are consistent with the AHA Life's Simple 7. These include four health behaviors—nonsmoking, increased physical activity, a healthy diet consistent with AHA guidelines, and a body mass index of <25 kg/m². Three ideal health factors were also included: an untreated blood pressure of less than 120/80 mm/Hg, untreated cholesterol of less than 200 mg/dL, and fasting blood sugar less than 100 mg/dL.

In addition, the Presidential Advisory incorporated the importance of continuing social engagements and also recognized that bodily functions such as sleep, stress, and appetite are also affected by the brain.

The concept of defining "optimal" brain health is to help physicians include these factors in discussions with their patients. The goal is to help individuals achieve optimal capacity to function throughout the lifespan and optimize both cognitive capacity and also emotional status. The central role that physical activity plays in optimal brain health recognizes its importance in this area. More detail about physical activity and its effects on the brain can be found in Chapter 11.

2.17   SAFETY DURING PHYSICAL ACTIVITY

It is important to minimize the likelihood of adverse events when people are involved in physical activity. Typically, adverse events are relatively minor during physical activity and the benefits of increased physical activity far outweigh the potential of adverse events. Nonetheless, certain precautions are important to minimize adverse events. Not only can adverse events be uncomfortable and perhaps even life-threatening, but they may hinder the ability of a person to stick with a physical activity program.

Some of the parameters for improving the safety of physical activity include the following:

- Type of activity—Non-contact activities such as walking, swimming, and gardening are very low-risk activities. Activities where there are collisions or frequent contact with other people or the ground such as football, ice hockey, even basketball, or soccer have an increased risk of adverse events.
- Volume—The risk of injury is also related to the volume of physical activity. For example, swimmers who engage in excessively long workout are prone to more injuries as are runners who participate in a high number of miles per week.
- Progression—An increased risk of injuries is also related to excessive, rapid changes in volume of physical activity. For this reason, it is important to recommend to patients to start slowly and progress slowly. This will be handled in subsequent chapters related to physical activity prescription.

2.18   PROMOTION OF PHYSICAL ACTIVITY

Despite abundant evidence that regular physical activity yields multiple health benefits, a significant minority of individuals in the United States do not participate in physical activity on a regular basis. For this reason it is important to determine effective methodologies for promoting physical activity. These can involve individuals, community, or national initiatives as well as public policy and built environment issues. An enormous amount of research has gone into this area and this will be covered in greater detail in Chapter 20.

2.19 CONCLUSIONS

The benefits of increased physical activity are huge and span every stage of life. These benefits contribute to improved health and lower the risk of various chronic diseases as well as serving as an adjunct to other components of treatment. For all of these reasons, physicians and other health-care workers should discuss increased physical activity in every patient they encounter. The key concepts set forth in this chapter are designed to make sure that counseling for physical activity is based on common understanding of concepts and terminologies.

CLINICAL APPLICATIONS

- This chapter provides a framework for understanding the core concepts of physical activity.
- Less than 40% of physicians typically discuss physical activity in clinical encounters.
- Physicians need to be knowledgeable about the core concepts in physical activity in order to adequately prescribe it for patients in the most effective and safe ways.
- Physical activity is one of the key components in the emerging field of lifestyle medicine that will help individuals improve both short- and long-term health and quality of life.

REFERENCES

1. Physical Activity Guidelines Advisory Committee. 2018 Physical Activity Guidelines Advisory Committee. 2018 Physical Activity Guidelines Advisory Committee Scientific Report. Washington, DC: U.S. Department of Health and Human Services; 2018.
2. Framingham Heart Study. https://www.framinghamheartstudy.org/ [Accessed January 8, 2020].
3. Centers for Disease Control and Prevention. Leading Causes of Death, 1900–1998. https://www.cdc.gov/nchs/data/dvs/lead1900_98.pdf [Accessed January 8, 2020].
4. U.S. Department of Health Education and Welfare General's Report on Health Promotion and Disease Prevention. Healthy People: The surgeon, 1979.
5. Lalonde M. 1974. *A New Perspective on the Health of Canadians*. Minister of Supply and Services Canada (Ottawa, ON).
6. Surgeon general's report on physical activity and health. 1996. *JAMA*. 1996;276:522
7. U.S. Department of Health and Human Services. 2008. Physical Activity Guidelines for Americans. https://health.gov/paguidelines/2008/ [Accessed January 8, 2020].
8. 2015–2020 Dietary Guidelines for Americans. 2015. 8th Edition. December 2015. Available at https://health.gov/dietaryguidelines/2015/guidelines/ [Accessed January 8, 2020].
9. Physical Activity Guidelines Advisory Committee. 2018. Physical Activity Guidelines Advisory Committee. *Integrating the Evidence*. U.S. Department of Health and Human Services (Washington, DC), 2018.

10. Kennedy M. What physicians need to know, do, and say to promote physical activity. In Lifestyle Medicine (3rd edition). ed. J. M. Rippe, M.D., 153–162. CRC Press (Boca Raton, FL), 2019.
11. Rippe J. Lifestyle Medicine. Blackwell Science, Inc. (London), 1999.
12. Rippe J. Lifestyle Medicine (3rd edition). CRC Press (Boca Raton, FL), 2019.
13. American Heart Association. Council on Lifestyle and Cardiometabolic Health. https://professional.heart.org/professional/MembershipCouncils/ScientificCouncils/UCM_322856_Council-on-Lifestyle-and-Cardiometabolic-Health.jsp [Accessed on January 9, 2020].
14. American College of Lifestyle Medicine. https://www.lifestylemedicine.org/ [Accessed on January 9, 2020].
15. Rippe J. Lifestyle medicine: the health promoting power of daily habits and practices. Am J Lifestyle Med. 12:499–512, 2018.
16. Sadarangani K, Hamer M, Mindell J, et al. Physical activity and risk of all-cause and cardiovascular disease mortality in diabetic adults from Great Britain: pooled analysis of 10 population-based cohorts. Diabetes Care. 2014;37:1016–1023.
17. Centers for Disease Control and Prevention, National Center for Health Statistics. National Health Interview Survey (NIH), 1997-2015: 2015 data release. https://www.cdc.gov/nchs/nhis/nhis_2015_data_release.htm [Accessed January 9, 2020].
18. American College of Sports Medicine. ACSM's Guidelines for Exercise Testing and Prescription. Lippincott, Williams and Wilkins (Philadelphia, PA), 2010.
19. Carlson S, Fulton J, Schoenborn C, et al. Trend and prevalence estimates based on the 2008 physical activity guidelines for Americans. Am J Prev Med. 2010;39:305–313.
20. Lloyd-Jones D, Hong Y, Labarthe D, et al. Defining and setting national goals for cardiovascular health promotion and disease reduction: the American heart association's strategic impact goal through 2020 and beyond. Circulation. 2010;121:586–613.
21. Gorelick P, Furie K, Iadecola C, et al. American heart association/American stroke association. Defining optimal brain health in adults: a presidential advisory from the American heart association/American stroke association. Stroke. 2017;48:e284–e303.

3 Physical Activity and Cardiovascular Disease Risk-Reduction and Treatment

KEY POINTS

- Cardiovascular disease (CVD) is by far the leading cause of morbidity and mortality in the United States and around the world.
- Lifestyle interventions are key components of recommendations from the American Heart Association (AHA) and other professional organizations to lower the risk of CVD.
- Regular physical activity has been repeatedly shown to lower the risk of CVD, coronary heart disease (CHD), hypertension, heart failure (HF), and diabetes.
- Assessment of levels of physical activity and recommendations for appropriate increases, if necessary, should be part of every appointment with physicians.
- Despite the overwhelming evidence that regular physical activity is a powerful tool for lowering the risk of CVD, only 25% of adults achieve levels of regular PA to meet minimum standards for the Centers for Disease Control and Prevention (CDC) of at least 150 minutes per week of moderate-intensity aerobic exercise or at least 75 minutes of vigorous exercise and muscle strengthening activities of at least two days a week.
- Unfortunately only 40% of physicians encounter with patients involve recommendation for increased physical activity.
- Recommendations for increased physical activity should be a component of every clinical visit.

3.1 INTRODUCTION

What each person does in their daily lives profoundly influences the likelihood of developing various chronic diseases and, in particular, cardiovascular disease (CVD) (1). Thousands of studies support the concept that a variety of lifestyle measures including physical activity, sound nutritional practices, maintaining a proper body weight, and avoiding tobacco products reduce the risk of CVD.

The strength of the scientific literature supporting the health-promoting impacts of positive daily habits and actions has been underscored by their inclusion in virtually every evidence-based clinical guideline for the prevention of metabolically related diseases. These principles are also incorporated in numerous documents and guidelines from the American Heart Association (AHA) (2, 3) and the American College of Cardiology (ACC) (4).

Unfortunately, despite the overwhelming evidence in support of positive lifestyle measures, it has been very difficult for individuals to incorporate these practices in their daily lives. While improvement in lifestyle measures has been cited as a major reason for reduction in the incidence of CVD in the past 20 years, enormous challenges remain. For example, between 1980 and 2000, mortality rates from CHD in the United States fell by more than 40% (5). Nonetheless, CVD remains the leading source of worldwide mortality.

In the United States, CVD results in more than 40% of annual mortality. While almost half of the reduction of CVD between 1980 and 2000 has been attributed to improvement in lifestyle-related risk factors such as increased physical activity, smoking cessation, and better control of cholesterol and blood pressure, it is important to recognize that increases in obesity and diabetes moved in the opposite direction. These increases in lifestyle related risk factors could potentially wipe out all the gains achieved by other lifestyle related risk factors unless progress can be made to reduce these negative trends (5).

Despite overwhelming evidence that lifestyle factors significantly affect the risk of developing CVD, it has been very difficult for patients to adopt these habits and practices in their daily lives. For example, when the AHA released its Strategic Plan for 2020 it reported that only 5% of individuals achieved "ideal" cardiovascular health that involved a series of lifestyle factors such as regular physical activity, sound nutrition, weight management, and avoidance of tobacco as well as some cardiovascular health-related factors such as control of cholesterol, blood pressure, and glucose (2).

In the past decade, the AHA and ACC have been leaders in promoting the power of lifestyle habits and practices as key factors in promoting cardiovascular health. For example, in the AHA Strategic Plan for 2020, the concept of "primordial" prevention (preventing risk factors from occurring in the first place) was introduced into the cardiovascular lexicon in addition to the context of "ideal" cardiovascular health (2). Moreover, the role of lifestyle factors is central to the AHA and ACC clinical practice guidelines issued in 2013 (4). The AHA program called "Simple 7" also relies largely on lifestyle factors to lower the risk of CVD (6).

Numerous lifestyle habits and practices influence the likelihood of developing CVD in general, and CHD in particular; however, this chapter will focus on the preeminent place of physical activity among these lifestyle factors. A recent extensive evidence-based review of this literature is contained in the 2018 Physical Activity Guidelines for Americans Advisory Committee Scientific Report 2018 (7). Evidence from this document will serve as an important evidence-based underpinning for the recommendations made in this chapter.

The current chapter will focus largely on physical activity and its effect to lower the risk of CVD. This is not intended to underestimate the importance of other factors; however, physical activity has been shown to be a very powerful modality for lowering the risk of CVD.

3.2   THE SCOPE OF THE PROBLEM

CVD is defined by the CDC to encompass CHD, stroke, hypertension, and HF. CVD accounts for over one in three deaths in the United States (8). Over 2,000 Americans die of some manifestation of CVD every day—roughly one in every 40 seconds. Despite decades-long declines in CVD mortality, it remains the leading cause of death in the United States. It is estimated that over 600,000 Americans will have their first myocardial infarction (MI) this year and over 300,000 will be victims of a re-infarction (9). This means that Americans experience a coronary event every 34 seconds.

When those who are physically very active are compared to sedentary individuals, the risk of CHD is 150–240% higher in sedentary individuals (9). Sadly, only about 25% of Americans engage in enough exercise to meet minimum standards from the CDC and also the Physical Activity Guidelines for Americans (PAGA) 2018 of at least 150 minutes per week of moderate-intensity aerobic activity or at least 75 minutes of vigorous physical and two sessions of strength training activities (10). It is essential to note, and often misunderstood, that even a small amount of physical activity substantially lowers the risk of mortality in general and from CVD, in particular.

As illustrated in Figure 3.1, the steepest part of reduction of risk comes from individuals who were previously sedentary and begin to engage in physical activity of as little as 30 minutes per week (7).

As emphasized in Figure 3.1 taken from PAGA 2018, there is no lower threshold for benefit! Increasing benefits occur for individuals who engage in approximately 150 minutes of regular physical activity. Although meaningful benefits occur in individuals who engage in physical activity even substantially more than this. As illustrated in Figure 3.1, 70% of the benefit is achieved by individuals who engage in moderate physical activity such as walking approximately 30 minutes five times per week; however, 20% of the benefit occurs for individuals who accumulate only 30 minutes per week!

While only approximately 25% of individuals achieve the guideline of 150 minutes of moderate-intensity physical activity on a weekly basis, according to the CDC fewer than half adults meet even minimum recommendations of physical activity. The statistics for young people are even more alarming with fewer than 20% of adolescents performing the recommended 60 minutes or more of daily physical activity (11).

Despite the well-established benefits of regular physical activity, it is clear that many physicians are not encouraging their patients to exercise. For example, a survey of 175 primary care physicians revealed that only 12% were aware of the recommendations of the ACSM about physical activity (12). Another survey of 51 internal medicine residents showed that while 88% were confident in their knowledge of the benefits of exercise, only 25% demonstrated adequate knowledge useful for patient counseling (13). Since over 70% of the adult population visits their primary care physician on at least an annual basis, this constitutes a significant missed opportunity to educate people on a number of positive lifestyle habits in general and physical activity in particular.

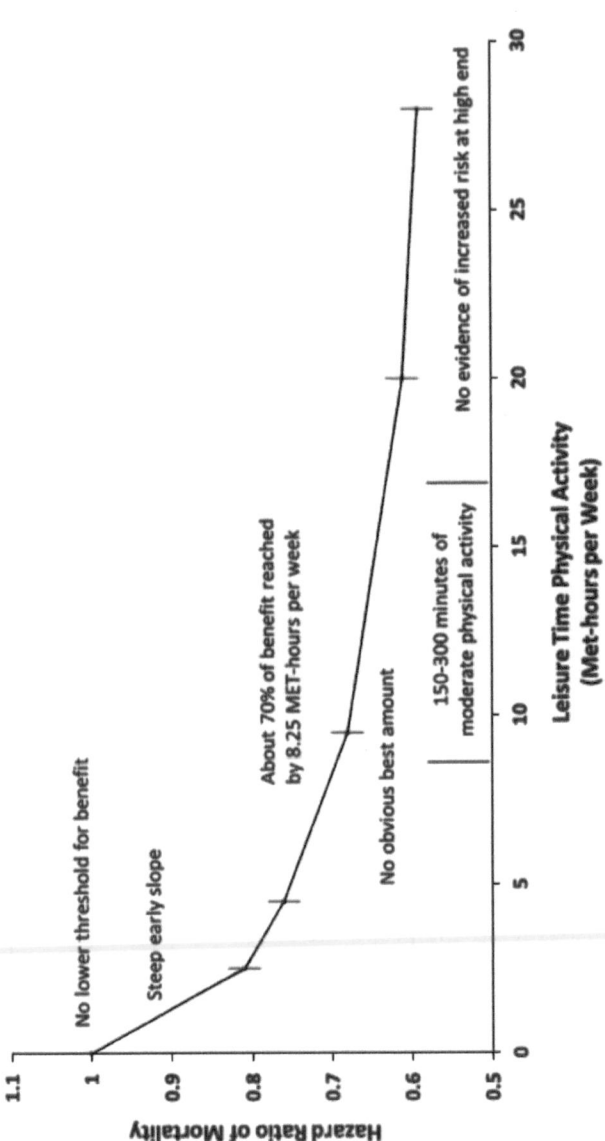

FIGURE 3.1　Relationship of moderate to vigorous physical activity to all-cause mortality with highlighted characteristics common to studies of this type. (From All-Cause Mortality. Cardiovascular Mortality and Incident Cardiovascular Disease. Part F. Chapter 6 in 2018 Physical Activity Guidelines Advisory Committee. 2018 Physical Activity Guidelines Advisory Committee. 2018 Physical Activity Committee Scientific Report. Washington, DC, US Department of Health and Human Services, 2018.)

3.3   PHYSICAL FITNESS VERSUS PHYSICAL ACTIVITY

A variety of techniques are utilized to measure both physical fitness and physical activity. The most accurate measurement of physical fitness involves the measurement of oxygen uptake (VO_2) during sustained activity. Tests of physical fitness are typically performed either on a treadmill or cycle ergometer. There are other physical fitness tests available using submaximal or indirect measures but these are less accurate. (These are discussed in more detail in Chapter 13.)

In contrast, physical activity is typically assessed by retrospective self-reported data (i.e. physical activity questionnaires). To further complicate matters, the definition of physical activity may vary considerably from study to study. ACSM defines moderate physical activity as any activity requiring 50–70% of VO_2 max or maximal heart rate (14). Vigorous physical is anything greater than 70% of VO_2 max or maximal heart rate. It is important to note that a specific activity such as brisk walking may not be enough to constitute even moderate physical activity for regular exercisers or healthy college-aged students whereas it could be vigorous physical activity for sedentary individuals or those over the age of 65.

It is also important to note that physical fitness may only be modestly correlated with physical activity. Correlations between 0.09 and 0.60 between physical fitness and physical activity have been found in various studies (15, 16). The most important finding is that reduction and risk of CHD or CVD is most strongly associated within individuals above the 25th percentile of physical fitness. Individuals below the 25th percentile of physical fitness have significantly increased at-risk by CHD by as much as 40%. This suggests that the greatest benefit for either physical activity or physical fitness occurs in the most sedentary population although additional benefits accrue to individuals above the 25th percentile level of physical fitness in a dose-response manner.

3.4   RECOMMENDATIONS FOR PHYSICAL ACTIVITY

A number of organizations have issued evidence-based guidelines for increasing physical activity. The guidelines include those from the PAGA 2008 (17) and 2018 (7) as well as the Surgeon General's Report for Physical Activity and Health (18) and the Practice Guidelines from AHA and ACC (4).

While there are slight differences in recommendations from these organizations, widespread agreement exists that some physical activity is better than none. Furthermore, the steepest part of the benefit curve with regard to reduction of risk of heart disease comes from those people who were truly sedentary who escape the bottom 20% of individuals in terms of physical activity and physical fitness. Here are some of the key concepts of recommendations from various organizations:

3.4.1   ADULTS

- Some activity is better than none. Adults who participate in any amount of physical activity (even as low as 30 minutes per week) gain some health benefits.
- Adults should optimally strive for at least 150 minutes per week of moderate-intensity physical activity or 75 minutes a week of vigorous intensity

physical activity or some combination of the two levels of activity. These individuals achieve approximately 70% reduction of risk of CVD.

- Additional reductions of risk of CVD can be obtained by exceeding 150 minutes of physical activity per week but the steepest part of the benefit curve comes for individuals who obtain 150 minutes a week of physical activity (approximately 30 minutes, five times a week).
- Muscle strengthening activities should be performed two or more days per week, which will result in additional risk reduction and health benefits.

3.4.2   Children and Adolescents

- Children and adolescents should perform 60 minutes of physical activity daily.
- Most of this activity should be moderate or vigorous-intensity aerobic physical activity.
- Vigorous physical activity should be performed at least three days a week.
- Young people should be encouraged to participate in physical activities appropriate for their age that are enjoyable and offer variety.

3.4.3   Older Adults

- Individuals over the age of 65 can also achieve significant health benefits from any amount of physical activity.
- Older adults who have chronic health conditions who cannot perform 150 minutes of moderate-intensity aerobic physical activity on a weekly basis should try to be as physically active as their conditions and abilities allow.
- Older adults should perform exercises that improve balance to lower their risk of falling.
- Older adults should determine their level of effort for physical activity relative to their level of fitness.
- Older adults with chronic conditions should understand how their conditions affect their ability to do regular physical activity safely. Consultation with a health-care professional may assist in this process.

3.5   STROKE

Stroke is an important component of overall CVD. It is estimated that 795,000 people in the United States experience either a new (approximately 610,000) or recurrent (approximately 185,000) stroke each year (1). Most of these strokes are ischemic (approximately 87%) and the remainder are hemorrhagic in nature. Certain groups are at higher risk for stroke. These include African Americans (nearly double the risk compared to Caucasians) who also tend to have strokes at a younger age. Hispanics and particularly Mexican Americans also have significantly higher rates of ischemic strokes, which also occur at a younger age than Caucasians. Additionally, 55,000 more women than men have strokes. The incidence of stroke in women aged 45–54 years old is especially high.

Transient Ischemic Attacks (TIAs) increase the risk of stokes both in the short- and long-term. There are between 200,000 and 500,000 TIAs in the United States each year (1). Approximately 15% of all strokes are preceded by a TIA. Approximately 12–13% of individuals will die within an year of a TIA.

The most significant risk factors for stroke include a history of TIA, pre-existing CHD, age, hypertension, diabetes, type 2 diabetes (T2DM), cigarette smoking, and atrial fibrillation.

Meta-analyses have shown that a reduction of risk of stroke associated with physical activity/aerobic exercise ranges between 20% and 40% (19, 20). The benefit for women is less clear and may not be as great as it is for men. The AHA currently recommends physical activity of at least 30 minutes per day of moderate-intensity physical activity to reduce the risk of ischemic stroke (21). There is some evidence that regular muscular strength training in younger individuals may modestly decrease the risk of stroke (5–10%), although the association has not been fully explored.

Inactivity has been shown to increase the risk of stroke and stroke mortality (1). However, its relationship to cerebral events is less well understood than CHD.

3.6   BRAIN HEALTH

Over the past decade, there has been an increased emphasis on brain health and its relationship to CVD. This is the underlying rationale for the joint initiative from the AHA and the American Stroke Association (ASA) with their campaign for "Optimal Brain Health" (22). The recommendations in this joint ASA/AHA initiative for physical activity and other forms of lifestyle practices and their impact on brain health are similar to the recommendations for lowering the risk of CVD. More on this topic will be discussed in Chapter 11.

3.7   HYPERTENSION

Hypertension is a well-established risk factor for CVD morbidity and mortality. Lifestyle modalities in general and physical activity in particular are well-established modalities for both prevention and treatment of high blood pressure. This fact has been incorporated in both the Joint National Commission (JNC) VII on Detection and Treatment of High Blood Pressure (23) and JNC VIII guidelines (24), as well as the 2017 ACC/AHA Guidelines for the Prevention, Detection, Evaluation, and Management of High Blood Pressure in Adults (25). The 2017 ACC/AHA guidelines established the classification and treatment thresholds detailed in Table 3.1. These guidelines also recommend a variety of non-pharmacologic interventions prominently featuring physical activity consisting of 120–150 minutes per week of aerobic physical activity and 90–120 minutes per week of dynamic resistance exercise.

The guidelines for blood pressure in the 2017 ACC/AHA recommendations were significantly lower than previous recommendations and were based on the findings of Systolic Blood Pressure Intervention Trial (SPRINT) (26). This trial was conducted in over 9,000 individuals with a mean age of 67.9 and a systolic blood pressure of 130–180 mm/Hg and at increased risk of cardiovascular events. The researchers compared targets of SBP < 120 mmHg to standard targets of

TABLE 3.1
Categories of Blood Pressure in Adults

BP Classification	Systolic Blood Pressure (SBP)	Diastolic Blood Pressure (DBP)	Lifestyle Habits	Drug Treatment	
Normal	BP	<120 mmHg	<80 mmHg	Promote	None
Elevated BP	120–129 mmHg	<80 mmHg	Yes	None	
Stage 1 hypertension	130–139 mmHg	80–89 mmHg	Yes	May be indicated*	
Stage 2 hypertension	>=140 mmHg	>=90 mmHg	Yes	Indicated+	

* =initiate pharmacological treatment if clinical atherosclerotic cardiovascular disease (ASCVD) or estimated 10 year CVD risk >10%.
+ Consideration of two medications from two different classes
Source: Adapted from 2017 ACC/AHA: Categories of BP in Adults

SBP<140 mmHg. The SPRINT trial showed a 30% decrease in the composite outcome of MI, acute coronary syndrome, stroke, and HF, or death compared to the standard target group. Unfortunately, in order to achieve these lower levels, three antihypertensive medicines were required in many participants, which may make it impractical in a normal clinical setting.

Numerous studies have reported an inverse association with leisure time physical activity and physical fitness and the development and severity of hypertension. The effects of regular physical activity on blood pressure levels have been established in over 70 randomized controlled trials and over 15 meta-analyses. In general, these studies have shown that moderate-intensity physical activity of 30–60 minutes per session three times per week conducted for 12–16 weeks lowers blood pressure in normotensive individuals, 2.6–4.7 mmHg in systolic, and 1.8–3.1 mmHg in diastolic blood pressure and reduction of systolic to 6–10 mmHg and diastolic blood pressure to 2.4–7.6 mmHg in patients with diagnosis of hypertension (27). Based on these data that moderate intensity (40–70% of maximal aerobic capacity) exercise sessions of three to five days per week is recommended as a highly effective component in prevention and management of high blood pressure (28, 29).

Resistance strength training has also been reported to result in reduction of blood pressure to approximately 7 mmHg systolic BP and 6 mmHg diastolic BP in some studies (30). However, not all studies have shown this level of reduction.

3.8 LIPIDS

The role of blood lipids in the pathology of atherosclerosis is well established (31). Dyslipidemia has been shown to be an important contributing factor to CHD. There are multiple components of dyslipidemia including elevation of total cholesterol (TC), low-density lipoprotein cholesterol (LDL-C), and triglycerides (TGs) as well as low levels of high-density cholesterol (HDL-C). Newer lipoprotein measures such as lipoprotein particle size and number of apolipoproteins as well as TG rich lipoproteins are also emerging as risk factors that may increase CVD risk (32).

The AHA and National Cholesterol Education Program (NCEP) Treatment Panel III have published guidelines establishing lipid and lipoprotein modification as important to both primary and secondary prevention (31).

The relationship between physical activity and lipids is complex (33). A number of cross- sectional studies have established that the volume and intensity of physical activity are related to increases in HDL-C levels and negatively associated with TG levels (34). The literature is, however, inconsistent on other blood lipids and physical activity. These findings are confounded by changes in body weight and body composition. In studies that explore physical activity but not dietary intervention, the most commonly reported change in lipids is an increase in HDL averaging 4.6% with simultaneous reductions of TG (3.7%) and LDL-C (5%) but not TC (34). Based on these findings regular physical activity cannot be recommended as a first line strategy for lowering TC or LDL-C.

It is important to note, however, that regular exercise may possibly have impact on components of the metabolic syndrome (see Section 3.9) that is strongly associated with the risk of CVD. There is little evidence that resistance strength training improves lipids.

3.9   METABOLIC SYNDROME

The clustering of established risk factors for CVD has been recognized for decades (35, 36). Most CVD occurs in people who have two or more established risk factors.

The metabolic syndrome represents a clustering of risk factors and is strongly linked to CVD as well as T2DM. Though there are a variety of definitions of metabolic syndrome, the one that is most commonly used, the AHA and National Heart, Lung and Blood Institute (NHLBI), utilizes the definition of metabolic syndrome from the NCEP, which requires that three of the following five criteria be present for the diagnosis of metabolic syndrome.

1. Impaired fasting glucose (IFG) represented by a fasting blood sugar ≥ 100 mg/dL
2. HDL-C < 40 mg/dL in men and < 50 mg/dL in women
3. TGs ≥ 150 mg/dL
4. Increased waist circumference ≥ 102 cm in men or ≥ 88 cm in women
5. Blood pressure ≥ 130/85 mmHg

It has been estimated that 36–38% of individuals in the United States have metabolic syndrome by these criteria (37). Unfortunately these same data suggest a 10% increase in the prevalence of metabolic syndrome in adults in the United States between 1988 and 2002. The increase in metabolic syndrome correlates with increase in prevalence of obesity and T2DM.

The association between physical activity and the prevalence of metabolic syndrome is not completely clear (38). Most of the cross-sectional studies have suggested that physical activity lowers both the prevalence and risk of metabolic syndrome but there appear to be a number of confounding factors such as gender, age, education, socioeconomic status as well as other risk factors such as smoking. Several longitudinal studies have suggested that increased physical activity particularly of vigorous intensity dramatically reduces the risk of developing metabolic syndrome. For example, one study showed that individuals who participated in 20 weeks of vigorous exercise for 30 minutes three times a week resulted in a decreased prevalence of metabolic syndrome by 30% (39).

There also appears to be a relationship between cardiorespiratory fitness and metabolic syndrome although this has not been studied as extensively as physical activity. In one study, individuals with low fitness (VO_2 max < 29.1 ml/kg per minute) were seven times more likely to have metabolic syndrome compared to individuals with a VO_2 max ≥ 35.5 ml/kg per minute. Several other studies have showed similar findings. The findings appeared to hold for women as well as men. It should be noted that increases in aerobic fitness may require more vigorous physical activity than moderate levels (38).

3.10   HEART FAILURE

It has been estimated that 5.7 million Americans suffer from HF (also known as congestive heart failure) (1). The risk of HF increases with age. By the time either a man or women reaches the age of 40 they a 20% lifetime risk of HF (1).

There have been very few studies that examine the relationship between physical activity and prevention of HF. Two large longitudinal studies compared sedentary individuals to those engaging in regular vigorous exercise and showed that those who exercised vigorously had a 15–35% low risk of developing HF (40, 41). Moderate-intensity physical activity has also been shown to decrease the risk of HF in individuals who participate in more than 4 hours a week of moderate activity such as walking, cycling, or swimming who have approximately 15% reduction in the lifetime risk of developing HF (40).

3.11   DIABETES

According to National Health and Nutrition Examiniation Survey (NHANES) data, 12.8% of Americans over the age of 19 have diabetes mellitus (DM) (1). Of these, greater than 90% are classified as T2DM. Furthermore, over 35% of Americans have been classified as pre-diabetic showing either impaired fasting glucose (IFG) or impaired glucose tolerance (1). This means that 47% of all adults in the United States have some degree of abnormal glucoregulation!

Diabetes is a significant risk factor for CHD. It is estimated that as many as 55% of adult diabetics have CHD (42, 43). T2DM is an independent risk factor for both MI and CHD in both men and women. Compared to non-diabetics, mortality from CHD has been estimated as two times greater in diabetic men and 4–5 times greater in diabetic women compared to non-diabetic controls. CVD is responsible for at least two-thirds of deaths in adults with DM. Diabetes is an important area where physical activity plays a significant role. This will be handled in Chapter 5.

3.12   OBESITY

Obesity is an independent risk factor for CVD and also is associated with multiple other risk factors or CVD including dyslipidemia and hypertension (44). The overall prevalence of overweight or obesity in the United States according to recent data is

69% in US adults (73% of men and 65% of women) (1). Overweight is considered as a body mass index (BMI) between 25 and 30 kg/m^2; obesity is any BMI greater than 30 kg/m^2.

It has become increasingly apparent that excess abdominal adipose tissue carries unique metabolic properties and may be more predictive of CVD, the metabolic syndrome, and diabetes than BMI or other measures of overall adiposity (45, 46).

Despite the high prevalence of overweight and its relationship to multiple other risk factors, unfortunately, less than 40% of obese adults were advised to lose weight by their family physician in 2004 compared to 42.3% in 1994 (47, 48). Furthermore, only slightly more than half of obese children were identified as such by their primary care physicians (49). Though physical activity alone is not a powerful way of helping individuals lose weight acutely, it is critically important for the long-term maintenance of weight loss.

Increased body weight and low levels of physical activity or fitness are associated with increased mortality from both CVD and T2DM. It has been argued, however, that overweight or obese individuals who have moderately high levels of fitness can ameliorate the increased risk of their excess weight. One extensive review in this debate, which has been called "Fit versus Fat," concluded that a physically active lifestyle and or moderately high fitness level (not in the bottom 20% of the population) reduces the risk of CVD/CHD in overweight or obese individuals (49) such that these individuals carry comparable risk associated with lean unfit persons. It has also been concluded, however, that the risk of these individuals is still greater than those who are fit and active and maintain a healthy weight. The issues related to physical activity and obesity are extremely important and will be handled in more detail in Chapter 10.

3.13   WOMEN AND HEART DISEASE

CVD is the leading cause of death in women in the United States. One in three women have some form of CVD and over 6.6 million women have been diagnosed with CHD (1). In the year 2013, 398,086 women died of CVD, about one death every 80 seconds (1). On average, new or recurrent MI as well as fatal CHD impact over 400,000 women in the United States each year. Unfortunately, since women typically have heart attacks at an older age than that of men they are more likely to die from them within a few weeks (1). Despite these startling statics, studies have indi cated that over 40% of women still do not know that CHD is by far the number one killer of women in the United States (1).

Regular physical activity has been demonstrated to significantly reduce the risk of CVD in women. Yet, fewer women (only 46.1%) compared to men (54.2%) engage in moderate to vigorous physical activity for three or more days a week (50). A number of cohort studies have shown that there is a dose/response relationship between physical activity and risk of CVD in both men and women. Data from the Women's Health Study showed that walking 1–1.5 hours per week was associated with 51% decrease in the risk of CVD (51). A 2004 meta-analysis of 30 longitudinal studies examining the impact of physical activity on the risk of CVD in women showed that there was a 20–40% reduction of risk of CVD in the most active women compared to those who are sedentary. A recent study of 17,000 older women in the Women's Health Study using accelerometer data showed a clear dose/response relationship between time engaged in "moderate" to "vigorous" physical activity and risk of CVD (52). The most active women had mortality rates 65% lower than women who were sedentary (53). It now appears that very similar benefits from ongoing physical activity in terms of reduction of CVD exist for both men and women.

3.14   CONCLUSION

CVD is by far the leading threat to health and longevity in both men and women in the United States and the world. The major risk factors for CVD are well known and the reduction of these risk factors can play a very important role in the prevalence of CHD, stroke, hypertension, and HF. Greater physical activity has been repeatedly shown to be a critically important modality for risk factor reduction in all forms of CVD. For all these reasons, it is incumbent upon physicians to inquire about levels of physical activity and, if found lower than optimal, prescribe ways of increasing it.

CLINICAL APPLICATIONS

- Every medical encounter should include assessment and recommendations for physical activity.
- Levels of physical activity should be geared to the age and current level of physical activity and fitness for each patient.
- Moderate-intensity physical activity at the level to help patients escape the bottom 20%, in terms of physical activity and physical fitness, results in the steepest part of the benefit curve for reduction of risk for CVD.

REFERENCES

1. Rippe J Lifestyle strategies for risk reduction, prevention and treatment of cardiovascular disease. Am J Lifestyle Medicine. 2018;13(2), 204–212.
2. Lloyd-Jones D, Hong Y, Labarthe D, et al. Defining and setting national goals for cardiovascular health promotion and disease reduction: the American Heart Association's strategic impact goal through 2020 and beyond. Circulation. 2010;121:586–613.
3. Chiuve S, McCullough M, Sacks F, et al. Healthy lifestyle factors in the primary prevention of coronary heart disease among men: benefits among users and nonusers of lipid-lowering and antihypertensive medications. Circulation. 2006;2:160–167.
4. Eckel R, Jakicic J, Ard J, et al. American College of Cardiology/American heart association task force on practice G. 2013 AHA/ACC guidelines on lifestyle management to reduce cardiovascular risk: a report of the American College of Cardiology/American heart association task force on practice guidelines. J Am Coll Cardiol. 2014;63:2960–2984.
5. Ford E, Ajani U, Croft J, et al. Explaining the decrease in U.S. deaths from coronary disease, 1980–2000. N Engl J Med. 2007;356:2388–2398.
6. AHA Simple 7. https://www.heart.org/en/professional/workplace-health/lifes-simple-7 [Accessed January 8, 2020].

7. Physical Activity Guidelines for Americans 2018. Internet. https://health.gov/paguidelines/second-edition/pdf/Physical_Activity_Guidelines_2nd_edition.pdf [Accessed January 8, 2020].

8. Writing Group, Mozaffarian D, Benjamin EJ, Go AS, et al. Heart disease and stroke statistics – 2016 update: a report from the American Heart Association. Circulation. 2016;133:e38–360.

9. Moore SC, Patel AV, Matthews CE. Leisure time physical activity of moderate to vigorous intensity and mortality: a large pooled cohort analysis. PLoS Med. 2012;9(11):e1001335–10.1371/journal.pmed.1001335. 10.1371/journal.pmed.1001335.

10. Adult participation in aerobic and muscle-strengthening physical activities—United States, 2011. MMWR. 2013;62 (17) 326–330.

11. Youth Risk Behavior Surveillance System. Internet. https://www.cdc.gov/healthyyouth/data/yrbs/index.htm [Accessed January 7, 2020].

12. Walsh JM, Swaganard DM, Davis T, et al. Exercise counseling by primary care physicians in the era of managed care. Am J Prev Med. 1999;16:307–313.

13. Rogers LQ, Gutin B, Humphries MC, et al. Evaluation of internal medicine residents as exercise role models and associations with self-reported counseling behavior, confidence, and perceived success. Teach Learn Med. 2006;18:215–221.

14. American College of Sports Medicine. ACSM's Guidelines for Exercise Testing and Prescription. Lippincott, Williams and Wilkins (Philadelphia PA), 2010.

15. Myers J, Kaykha A, George S, et al. Fitness versus physical activity patterns in predicting mortality in men. Am J Med. 2004;117:912–918.

16. Jacobs DR Jr, Ainsworth BE, Hartman TJ, et al. A simultaneous evaluation of 10 commonly used physical activity questionnaires. Med Sci Sports Exerc. 1993;25:81–91.

17. US Department of Health and Human Services. 2008. Physical Activity Guidelines 2008. Internet. https://health.gov/paguidelines/2008/ [Accessed January 8, 2020].

18. Physical Activity and Health: A Report of the Surgeon General. U.S. Department of Health and Human Services. Centers for Disease Control and Prevention. July 11, 1996.

19. Reimers C, Knapp G, Reimers A. Exercise as stroke prophylaxis. Dtsch Arztebl Int. 2009;106:715–721.

20. Lee C, Folsom A, Blair S. Physical activity and stroke risk: a meta-analysis. Stroke. 2003;34:2475–2481.

21. Goldstein L, Bushnell C, Adams R, et al. Guidelines for the primary prevention of stroke: a guideline for healthcare professionals from the American Heart Association/American Stroke Association. Stroke. 2011;42:517–584.

22. Gorelick P, Furie K, Iadecola C, et al. Defining optimal brain health in adults: a presidential advisory from the American Heart Association/American Stroke Association. Stroke. 2017;48:e284–e303.

23. Chobanian A, Bakris G, Black H, et al. The Joint National Committee on prevention, detection, evaluation and treatment of high blood pressure. The Seventh Report of the Joint National Committee on Prevention, Detection, Evaluation, and Treatment of High Blood Pressure: The JNC 7 Report. JAMA. 2003;289:2560–2572.

24. James P, Oparil S, Carter BL, et al. 2014 Evidence-based Guideline for the Management of High Blood Pressure in Adults: Report from the panel members appointed to the Eighth Joint National Committee (JNC 8). JAMA. 2014;311:507–520.

25. Whelton P, Carey R, Aronow W, et al. 2017 ACC/AHA/AAPA/ABC/ACPM/AGS/APHA/ASH/ASPC/NMA/PCNA Guideline for the Prevention, Detection, Evaluation, and Management of High Blood Pressure in Adults: A Report of the American College of Cardiology/American Heart Association Task Force on Clinical Practice Guidelines. Hypertension. 2018;71:e13–e115.

26. SPRINT Research Group, Wright J, Jr., Williamson J, Whelton P, et al. A randomized trial of intensive versus standard blood-pressure control. N Engl J Med. 2015;373:2103–2116.

27. 2018 Physical Activity Guidelines Advisory Committee. 2018 Physical Activity Guidelines Advisory Committee Scientific Report. Washington, DC: U.S. Department of Health and Human Services, 2018. Individuals with Chronic Conditions. Part F. Chapter 10.

28. Kukkonen K, Rauramaa R, Voutilainen E, et al. Physical training of middle-aged men with borderline hypertension. Ann Clin Res.1982;14 Suppl 34:139–145.

29. Leon A, Casal D, Jacobs D. Effects of 2,000 kcal per week of walking and stair climbing on physical fitness and risk factors for coronary heart disease. J Cardiopulm Rehabil. 1996;16:183–192.

30. Cornelissen VA, Fagard RH. Effect of resistance training on resting blood pressure: a meta-analysis of randomized controlled trials. J Hypertens. 2005;23:251–259.

31. Grundy S, Cleeman J, Merz C, et al. Implications of recent clinical trials for the National Cholesterol Education Program Adult Treatment Panel III Guidelines. J Am Coll Cardiol. 2004;44:720–732.

32. Tóth PP, Potter D, Ming EE. Prevalence of lipid abnormalities in the United States: The National Health and Nutrition Examination Survey 2003–2006. J Clin Lipidol. 2012;6:325–330.

33. 2018 Guidelines on the Management of Blood Cholesterol. Internet. https://www.acc.org/~/media/Non-Clinical/Files-PDFs-Excel-MS-Word-etc/Guidelines/2018/Guidelines-Made-Simple-Tool-2018-Cholesterol [Accessed January 8, 2020].

34. El Harchaoui K, Arsenault B, Franssen R, et al. High-density lipoprotein particle size and concentration and coronary risk. Ann Intern Med. 2009;150:84–93.

35. Bonora E. The metabolic syndrome and cardiovascular disease. Ann Med. 2006; 38:64–80.

36. Grundy SM, Brewer HB, Cleeman JI, et al. Definition of Metabolic Syndrome: Report of the National Heart, Lung, and Blood Institute/American Heart Association Conference on Scientific Issues Related to Definition. Circulation. 2004;109:433–438.

37. Ford E, Giles W, Dietz W. Prevalence of the metabolic syndrome among US adults: findings from the Third National Health and Nutrition Examination Survey. JAMA. 2002;287:356–359.

38. Churilla J, Zoeller R. Physical activity and the metabolic syndrome: a review of the evidence. Am J Lifestyle Med. 2008;2:118–125.

39. Grundy S, Cleeman J, Daniels S, et al. Diagnosis and management of the metabolic syndrome: an American heart Association/National Heart, Lung, and Blood Institute scientific statement. Circulation. 2005;112:2735–2752.

40. Kenchaiah S, Sesso HD, Gaziano JM. Body mass index and vigorous physical activity and the risk of heart failure among men. Circulation. 2009;119:44–52.

41. Hu G, Jousilahti P, Antikainen R, et al. Joint effects of physical activity, body mass index, waist circumference, and waist-to-hip ratio on the risk of heart failure. Circulation. 2010;121:237–44.

42. Hammoud T, Tanguay J, Bourassa MG. Management of coronary artery disease: therapeutic options in patients with diabetes. J Am Coll Cardiol. 2000;36:355–365.

43. Van de Werf F, Ardissino D, Betriu A, et al. Management of acute myocardial infarction in patients presenting with ST-segment elevation. Eur Heart J. 2003;24:28–66.

44. Poirier P, Giles T, Bray G, et al. Obesity and cardiovascular disease: pathophysiology, evaluation, and effect of weight loss – an update of the 1997 American Heart Association Scientific Statement on Obesity and Heart Disease from the Obesity Committee of the Council on Nutrition Physical Activity, and Metabolism. Circulation. 2006;113:898–918.

45. Bonora E. Relationship between regional fat distribution and insulin resistance. Int J Obes Relat Metab Disord. 2000;24 Suppl. 2:S32–S35.
46. Sharma AM. Adipose tissue: a mediator of cardiovascular risk. International J Obes. 2002;26 Suppl. 4:S5–S7.
47. Abid A, Galuska D, Khan LK, Gillespie C, Ford CS, Serdula MK. Are healthcare professionals advising patients to lose weight? A trend analysis. Med Gen Med. 2005;7:10.
48. O'Brien S, Holubkov R, Reis EC. Identification, evaluation, and management of obesity in an academic primary care center. Pediatrics. 2004;114:e154–e159.
49. Gill J, Malkova D. Physical activity, fitness and cardiovascular disease risk in adults: interactions with insulin resistance and obesity. Clin Sci. 2004;110:409–425.
50. Carlson S, Fulton J, Schoenborn C. Trend and prevalence estimates based on the 2008 Physical Activity Guidelines for Americans. Am J Prev Med. 2010;39:305–313.
51. Lee IM, Rexrode KM, Cook NR, et al. Physical activity and coronary heart disease in women: is "no pain, no gain" passé? JAMA. 2001;285:1447–1454.
52. Lee IM, Shiroma EJ, Evenson KR, et al. Accelerometer-measured physical activity and sedentary behavior in relation to all-cause mortality: the Women's Health Study. Circulation. 2018;137:203–205.

4 Physical Activity and the Prevention and Treatment of Cancer

KEY POINTS

- Numerous cancers are linked to an inactive lifestyle.
- Physical activity has been shown to play important and positive roles in lowering the risk of cancer in the first place and helping in its treatment if already present.
- The Physical Activity Guidelines for Americans 2018 Scientific Report has greatly expanded the literature on the number of cancers where there is strong evidence that increased physical activity can play multiple positive roles.
- Every clinician should discuss and prescribe physical activity to cancer patients through the entire spectrum of these diseases.
- Physicians should include reducing the risk of many cancers when they discuss the benefits of physical activity with all patients.

4.1   INTRODUCTION

Cancer is very prevalent in the United States and around the world. Nearly one in six deaths worldwide is attributable to cancer (1), which equates to 8.8 million deaths (2) annually. Over the next 20 years, the global cancer burden is expected to rise by 70%. As of 2016 over 15.5 million living Americans (approximately 4.8% of the population) have been diagnosed with cancer at some point in their lives (3, 4). In the United States, 1,688,780 new cancer cases and 600,920 cancer deaths were projected to occur in 2017 s(1).

On average 38% of American women and 48% of American men will be diagnosed with invasive cancer at some point in their lifetime (5). Though there are genetic causes of cancer, most cases of cancer are due to the environment or lifestyle (6). Physical activity, or lack thereof, plays an important role in the likelihood of developing cancer. Other known lifestyle and preventable causes of cancer include tobacco use, alcohol intake, diet, obesity, and behaviors that increase exposure to oncogenic viruses. In spite of the fact that all of these lifestyle factors are important, this chapter will focus on the critical role that physical activity plays in the reduction in the risk of cancer. Although there is also evidence that some childhood cancers may also be ameliorated by lifestyle factors, this chapter will focus on the role of physical activity in the prevention and treatment of cancer in adults.

In the decade between 2005 and 2015, a number of new cancer cases increased by 33% globally (7). The direct medical cost for cancer in 2014 in the United States surpassed $87.7 billion with 58% of the cost coming from office-based providers of hospital outpatient services and 27% due to inpatient hospital services.

With these compelling statistics it is important to develop efficacious, cost-effective strategies for preventive and therapeutic care for cancer. Physical activity represents one of the important lifestyle modalities that has been demonstrated to lower the risk of cancer as well as serve as an important adjunct to all phases of treatment of various malignancies.

4.2   THE ROLE OF PHYSICAL ACTIVITY IN CANCER PREVENTION

There is no longer any serious doubt that a healthy lifestyle plays an important role in the prevention and treatment of cancers (8, 9). Physical activity, in particular, plays a central role in the lifestyle prevention and treatment of cancer.

While exact mechanisms as to how physical activity results in cancer risk reduction are not completely understood, there is increasing documentation from the Physical Activity Guidelines for Americans 2018 and other evidence-based sources that regular physical activity plays a role in not only reducing the risk of cancer, but also various phases of its treatment. This includes primary prevention, which largely reflects risk reduction in healthy populations. Secondary prevention involves screening, detecting, diagnosing, and treating early stages of pre-malignant cancers. Tertiary treatment revolves around symptom management, rehabilitation, and end of life care. Physical activity can play an important role in all three of these levels.

Most research in the area of physical activity and specific cancers has focused on colon cancer, breast cancer, and/or endometrial cancer (8). However, an increasing number of cancers have been linked to inactivity. The World Cancer Research Fund International reported that 20% of cancer cases in the United States could be prevented by increased physical activity, weight control, and consumption of a healthy diet (6). In addition, 12 prospective cohort studies involving 1.44 million participants in the United States and Europe demonstrated an association between higher levels of physical activity and reduction of risk in 13 different cancers (9). The Physical Activity Guidelines for Americans Advisory Committee 2018 Scientific Report (1) listed multiple cancers where there is strong or moderate evidence that physical activity exerts a protective effect on lowering risk of these cancers. Specific cancers will be handled in more detail later in this chapter.

4.3   THE ROLE OF PHYSICAL ACTIVITY IN PRIMARY
CANCER PREVENTION

Approximately 12% of American women will develop invasive breast cancer during their lifetime. Over 40,000 women will die of breast cancer in the United States in 2017 (10–12). Research from over these three decades shows that inactivity has been associated with increased breast cancer risk. Physical activity has been particularly shown to be efficacious in breast cancer risk reduction in both pre- and postmenopausal women (13). Some studies have also suggested a relationship between inactivity and breast cancer in both postmenopausal women and premenopausal women. Although the role of physical activity in the reduction of breast cancer risk is not completely understood, it may be mediated by the reduction of sex hormones and increasing concentration of sex hormone binding globulin proteins (14). Regular exercise may also decrease adiposity and lower the overexpression of estrogen (15). These mechanisms related to the reduction of biologically available sex hormones may play a prominent role in decreasing not only the risk of breast cancer, but also endometrial, ovarian, prostate, and testicular cancers.

Inactivity has also been shown to correlate with increased colon cancer risk (16). The mechanism for risk factor of colon cancer reduction has been postulated to potentially relate to increased immune function and reductions in stool transit time, hyperinsulinemia, and inflammation (17, 18). Despite these postulates, the exact cause for reduction in the risk of colon cancer remains incompletely understood. Nonetheless, a recent study of non-diabetic patients revealed that physical activity is associated with a 20% reduced risk of colon cancers.

4.4 THE ROLE OF PHYSICAL ACTIVITY IN SECONDARY CANCER PREVENTION

Physical activity may also play a role once a cancer has been diagnosed. In particular, physical activity has been shown to reduce some of the effects of treatment for cancer including fatigue, anxiety, depression, and reduced sexual activity (19, 20). One recent review suggested that regular physical activity, such as brisk walking, resulted in fewer symptoms and side effects during treatment (21). Specifically, many patients identify physical activity as one of the most effective deterrents to fatigue (22).

In addition to lowering side effects of treatment, physical activity in cancer patients may also yield improvements in health status and long-term health outcomes. In one study of breast cancer patients' mortality decreased by 39% and overall mortality decreased by 46%, when the most active patients were compared to the least active (23). These findings are particularly important since it has been demonstrated that breast cancer patients may decrease total physical activity by up to two hours per week when comparing pre- and post-diagnosis (22).

With all of these considerations as background, clinicians should advocate physical activity as an important secondary treatment tool for both physical and psychological wellbeing of patients after the diagnosis of cancer.

4.5 THE ROLE OF PHYSICAL ACTIVITY IN TERTIARY CANCER TREATMENT

Physical activity can also serve as a valuable tool during rehabilitation and chronic disease management for cancer patients. In one analysis of 26 prospective cohort studies of breast, colorectal, and prostate cancer, a 37% pooled risk reduction of cancer-specific mortality was demonstrated when comparing most-active to least-active patients (24). Importantly, regular physical activity, when compared to other lifestyle factors such as smoking, diet, and alcohol intake, has been shown to have the strongest effect in attenuating the risk of breast cancer recurrence and reducing mortality. Physical activity has been shown to help patients increase longevity and quality of life (25). There are multiple, postulated mechanisms for the physical activity-mediated benefits in tertiary cancers. Regulation of inflammation and natural killer cell function may play a role.

Other mechanisms have been postulated in different cancer types, while others restricted to specific cancers. It is important to emphasize that physical activity is unique in generating only positive sequelae in cancer patients. There have been no studies that demonstrate that physical activity adversely affects cancer outcomes. It is, of course, imperative that clinicians take into account potential cancer-related side effects to appropriately modify exercise prescriptions and personalize prescriptions for both cancer and non-cancer patients.

4.6   CANCERS FOR WHICH PHYSICAL ACTIVITY SHOWS STRONG EVIDENCE OF PROTECTIVE EFFECTS

A comprehensive listing of the relationship between types of cancers where physical activity has shown strong evidence of protective effects has been summarized in the recently released 2018 PAGA Scientific Report (26). The reader is referred to this comprehensive document for further information. In this section, these findings will be briefly summarized by cancer type with the 2018 PAGA grading utilized.

- Bladder cancer—Strong evidence demonstrates that greater amounts of physical activities are associated with reduced risk of developing bladder cancer.
- Breast cancer—Strong evidence demonstrates that greater amounts of physical activities are associated with lower risk of breast cancer.
- Colon cancer—Strong evidence demonstrates that greater amounts of recreational, occupational, or total physical activities are associated with lower risk of developing colon cancer.
- Endometrial cancer—Strong evidence demonstrates that greater amounts of physical activities are associated with lower risk of endometrial cancer.
- Esophageal cancer—Strong evidence demonstrates that greater amounts of recreational, occupational or total physical activities are associated with lower risk of developing endocarcinoma of the esophagus.
- Gastric cancer—Strong evidence demonstrates that greater amounts of physical activities are associated with lower risk of developing gastric cancer.
- Renal cancer—Strong evidence demonstrates that greater amounts of physical activities are associated with reduced risk of developing renal cancer.
- Lung cancer—Moderate evidence demonstrates that greater amounts of physical activities are associated with lower risk of lung cancer.
- Hematologic cancer—Limited evidence suggests no relationship between physical activity and leukemia incidence. Limited evidence suggests that physical activity has a protective effect on lymphoma and myeloma risk such that greater amounts of physical activities reduce the risk of lymphoma and myeloma.
- Head and neck cancer—Limited evidence suggests that greater amounts of physical activities are associated with lower risk of head and neck cancer incidence.

- Ovarian cancer—Limited evidence suggests a weak relationship between greater levels of physical activities and lower risk of ovarian cancer.
- Pancreatic cancer—Limited evidence suggests that greater amounts of physical activities are associated with a lower risk of developing pancreatic cancer.
- Prostate cancer—Limited evidence suggests a weak relationship between greater levels of physical activities and lower prostate cancer risk.
- Brain cancer—Insufficient evidence is available to determine whether a relationship between physical activities and overall brain cancer incidence exists. Limited evidence suggests that physical activity decreases the risk of certain types of brain cancers, specifically a reduced risk is observed for glioma and meningioma.
- Thyroid cancer—Moderate evidence indicates that greater amounts of physical activities are not associated with risk of developing thyroid cancer.
- Rectal cancer—Limited evidence suggests that greater amounts of physical activities are not associated with risks of developing rectal cancer.

4.7 DEFINING "HEALTH-ENHANCING" PHYSICAL ACTIVITY FOR CANCER PATIENTS

A number of organizations have offered general guidance and recommendations for "health-enhancing" physical activity for cancer patients. The American College of Sports Medicine (ACSM) has offered numerous guidelines that have evolved to include physical activities as well as structured exercise programs for health-enhancing benefits in cancer patients (27).

With regard to physical activity and cancer, most clinicians now consider physical activity as an integral strategy for cancer primary prevention, secondary and third prevention, and tertiary prevention and treatment. Numerous physical activity guidelines for cancer patients have been released over the past decade outlining specific recommendations for physical activity and cancer patients (28).

Physical activity can help prevent some cancers and also can be utilized as a treatment for populations where cancer is already present. Both safety and efficacy are fundamental concerns surrounding physical activity and exercise among cancer survivors.

Guidelines from the American Cancer Society have been issued outlining the role of physical activity during treatment (29), recovery, and post diagnosis and life-long disease-free living. ACSM has recommended that individuals in remission with stable disease status should engage in regular physical activities for 150 minutes per week and include strength training exercises at least twice per week (27).

The American Institute for Cancer Research (AICR) has recommended daily physical activity for cancer survivors with the goal of 30 minutes of moderate intensity physical activity each day or 210 minutes per week to minimize the risk of cancer recurrence (30). The AICR also, in addition to aerobic activity, recommends incorporating strength training exercises at least two days per week. The National Comprehensive Cancer Network has recommended guidelines for individuals undergoing cancer treatment proposing 30 minutes of aerobic exercise at least five times per week (31). This regimen is aimed at lessening cancer-related fatigue. Thus, guidelines from various organizations all recommend physical activity for treating and decreasing the risk of reoccurrence of cancer.

4.8　PHYSICAL ACTIVITY, OVERWEIGHT, OBESITY, AND CANCER

Overweight and obesity are clearly associated with increased risk of developing many cancers including cancers of the breast in postmenopausal women, colon and rectum, endometrium and adenocarcinoma of the esophagus, kidney, and pancreas. Since overweight and obesity are endemic in the United States, many cancer survivors are overweight or obese at the time of diagnosis (32, 33).

In addition to reduction of energy intake, regular physical activity can play an important role in helping individuals lose weight and/or maintain a healthy body weight. Regular physical activity can also help individuals who are cancer survivors retain or regain muscle mass and promote the maintenance of weight loss in patients who are overweight or obese.

Throughout the cancer continuum, individuals should strive to achieve and maintain healthy body weight as defined by body mass index (BMI) between 18.5 kg/m^2 and 25 kg/m^2 (34, 35). Physical activity plays an important role in helping to maintain a healthy body weight. More detailed information concerning the links between overweight and obesity and cancer may be found in Chapter 10.

4.9　SEDENTARY BEHAVIOR AND CANCER INCIDENCE

The 2018 PAGA concluded that there was moderate evidence indicating a significant relationship between greater time spent in sedentary behavior and higher risk of cancer particularly endometrial, colon, and lung cancer (26). The PAGA 2018 reported that when comparing the highest levels to lowest levels of sedentary time, the increased risk of endometrial, colon, and lung cancers risk-reduction ranged from 20% to 35% (26).

4.10　PHYSICAL ACTIVITY GUIDELINES FOR CANCER PATIENTS

General guidelines for all phases of cancer prevention generally follow the recommendations from the ACSM and the 2018 PAGA Scientific Report. These include accumulation of 150 minutes of moderate intensity physical activity or 75 minutes of vigorous physical activity per week (29).

With regard to the cancer survivors, the American Cancer Society makes the following recommendations:

- Avoid inactivity and return to normal daily activities as soon as possible following diagnosis.
- Aim to exercise at least 150 minutes per week.

TABLE 4.1

Clinical Recommendations for Physical Activity

Organization	Target Population	Stage in Cancer Care Continuum	Recommendation
American Cancer Society	Adults	Prevention	150 mins. moderate intensity, 75 mins. vigorous intensity, or equivalent combination of the two each week [44]
American Cancer Society	Children	Prevention	60 mins. moderate or vigorous intensity each day; at least three days with vigorous intensity activity [44]
American Cancer Society	Nonspecific	Survivorship	150 mins. exercise with strength training activities at least twice per week [49]
American College of Sports Medicine	Adults	Prevention	30 mins. moderate to vigorous activity five times per week; at least two days of strength training each week [42]
American Institute for Cancer Research	Nonspecific	Prevention	30 mins. moderate activity every day; limit sedentary habits [43]
American Institute for Cancer Research	Nonspecific	Survivorship	30 mins. moderate intensity activity each day; at least two days of strength training each week [50]
Oncology Nursing Society	Nonspecific	Survivorship	150 mins. moderate intensity or 75 mins. vigorous intensity aerobic activity [51]
National Comprehensive Cancer Network	Nonspecific	Treatment	30 mins. aerobic activity at least five times per week [52]

From Keltner CH and Bowles HR. Physical Activity and the Prevention and Treatment of Cancer. In Rippe JM: Lifestyle Medicine, 3rd edition, CRC Press (Boca Raton), 2019. (Used with Permission of the editor of Lifestyle Medicine, Dr. James Rippe)

- Include strength training exercises at least two days per week.
- Achieve and maintain a healthy body weight by eliminating consumption of high calorie foods and beverages and increasing physical activity to promote weight loss if necessary.
- A summary of recommendations from various organizations with regard to physical activity and cancer patients may be found in Table 4.1.

4.11 PHYSICAL ACTIVITY GUIDELINES ADHERENCE

Adherence to regular physical activity is an important aspect of its utilization in cancer prevention and therapy. Since physical activity should be a central component of cancer prevention and treatment strategies, it is important to encourage consistent moderate to vigorous physical activity. Clinicians should recognize potential barriers to the achievement of regular physical activity in cancer patients, since behavior change is a significant component of adopting a regular physical activity program.

A number of aspects of cancer and its treatment can compromise the patient's ability to incorporate regular physical activity in their lives (36). Fatigue related to cancer or cancer treatment can impede physical functioning both during treatment and during remission. Conversely, several factors can increase the likelihood of adhering to physical activity such as pretreatment physical activity levels.

Pretreatment fatigue, emotional disturbances from treatment, and marital status, however, have been shown to also decrease the likelihood of adhering to physical activity programs (37, 38). Symptoms such as pain, fatigue, or malaise from symptoms and treatment can provide further obstacles to cancer patients' ability to engage in physical activity. Psychological and logistical constraints can also contribute to difficulty adhering to regular programs of physical activity. Time restriction based on physical examinations and other commitments as well as logistical limitations within hospitals can also further create barriers of physical activity in cancer patients (39).

Isolation and lack of motivation can also present unique challenges to cancer patients (40). For example, patients may believe that exercising around other severely ill patients may make them feel sicker, whereas others believe that maximizing sleep is the best way to reduce side effects of chemotherapy or similar treatments. Thus, it is important that clinicians employ various behavior based strategies to overcome some of these challenges.

4.12   STRATEGIES FOR PHYSICAL ACTIVITY INTERVENTIONS

Since multiple factors may contribute to barriers for cancer patients to achieve adequate physical activity, it is important that clinicians adopt strategies to meet the unique needs of each patient. Several studies have shown that self-efficacy is a powerful factor that increases adherence to physical activity (41, 42). Not only giving patients general advice about the importance of physical activity but also helping them determine which forms of physical activities are most likely to be enjoyable for them can enhance self-efficacy.

It is also important to recognize that many cancer survivors may have barriers such as time, money, and transportation. All of these should be addressed as practical considerations related to increasing the likelihood of physical activity adherence. The positive news is that patients with cancer have been shown to be highly receptive to counseling in the area of physical activity. In one study of cancer survivors aged 20–44, 78% were interested in participating in a physical activity program and 50% wanted to receive counseling in this area from their clinicians (43). Physical activity counseling from the nursing staff has also been shown to increase adherence among patients undergoing intensive cancer regimens (44).

Finally, the explosion of technologies may enhance the likelihood of engaging in physical activity programs (45, 46). Cancer patients should be directed to the wealth of materials that are now available on the internet as well as wearable technologies.

4.13   CANCER AS A METABOLIC DISEASE

A wealth of information on physical activity and other lifestyle factors is available on CVD and diabetes, which are clearly recognized as metabolic diseases. Cancer, however, should also be recognized as a metabolic disease. Many of the same recommendations that are given to lower the risk or help in the treatment of CVD and type 2 diabetes (T2DM) apply with minimal changes to patients with cancer. This is the underlying premise of the Joint Statement from the AHA/ACS/ADA on the Prevention and Treatment of CVD, T2DM, and cancer (47). In all three of these metabolically based diseases, components of positive lifestyle have been shown to be efficacious both in prevention and in treatment. Physical activity is one of the key recommendations that should be made to all patients who have any of these conditions.

4.14   FUTURE DIRECTIONS IN RESEARCH

While numerous studies have shown that physical activity is a powerful modality for cancer prevention and as a strategy for minimizing symptoms and maximizing quality of life and longevity in cancer patients, future research can clarify a number of issues. For example, the relationship between cancer risk and survivorship remains hampered by fundamental uncertainty regarding the underlying biological mechanisms involved in this linkage. This area is further complicated by the multi-factorial etiology of cancers—some of which are linked to sedentary lifestyle. This makes it difficult to separate the effects of physical activity from other health-promoting behaviors. In addition, since physical activity interacts with weight management, teasing out the benefits from the physical activity component may be quite challenging. Nonetheless, the bottom line remains that physical activity has been shown to be a powerful tool in every phase of many cancers.

4.15   CONCLUSIONS

Substantial evidence now exists to support inactivity as a major risk factor for multiple cancers and the value of increased physical activity to either lower the risk of cancer assisting in its treatment or ameliorate some of the symptoms. Thus, it is incumbent upon clinicians to discuss and prescribe physical activity for cancer patients at every level of this disease whether it be primary, secondary, or tertiary prevention and/or treatment.

CLINICAL IMPLICATIONS

- Clinicians should discuss the power of physical activity to lower the risk of cancers or ameliorate symptoms and progression of these conditions at every step along the spectrum of these diseases.
- Since cancer patients may have a unique set of barriers related to the likelihood of initiating and adhering to physical activity programs, these issues should be discussed in every clinical appointment.
- Though the exact biological mechanisms are not completely understood as to how physical activity beneficially impacts on reducing the risk of cancer and improving its treatment, the data from multiple cohort studies strongly suggest that physical activity plays an important role in preventing and treating cancer.

- While other risk factors such as poor diet, alcohol consumption, and tobacco utilization also impact on cancer risk, physical activity is the most powerful tool that clinicians have at their disposal to help individuals reduce their risk of cancer or help in its treatment.
- The interaction between physical activity and weight management underscores the importance of utilizing physical activity recommendations for cancer patients who are overweight or obese.

REFERENCES

1. Siegel R, Miller K, Jemal A. Cancer statistics, 2017. CA Cancer J Clin. 2017;67(1):7–30.
2. World Health Organization: Cancer: Key facts. http://www.who.int/mediacentre/factsheets/fs297/en/ [Accessed January 6, 2020].
3. American Cancer Society: Cancer Facts and Figures 2017. https://www.cancer.org/content/dam/cancer-org/research/cancer-facts-and-statistics/annual-cancer-facts-and-figures/2017/cancer-facts-and-figures-2017.pdf [Accessed January 6, 2020].
4. United States Census Bureau: QuickFacts: United States 2016. https://www.census.gov/quickfacts/table/PST045216/00 [Accessed January 6, 2020].
5. American Cancer Society. Lifetime risk of developing or dying from cancer. https://www.cancer.org/cancer/cancer-basics/lifetime-probability-of-developing-or-dying-fromcancer.html. Updated March 23, 2016 [Accessed January 6, 2020].
6. World Cancer Research Fund International: Cancer preventability estimates for diet, nutrition, body fatness, and physical activity. http://wcrf.org/int/cancer-facts-figures/preventability-estimates/cancer-preventability-estimates-diet-nutrition [Accessed January 6, 2020].
7. Global burden of disease cancer collaboration. Global, regional, and national cancer incidence, mortality, years of life lost, years lived with disability, and disability-adjusted life-years for 32 cancer groups, 1990 to 2015: a systematic analysis for the global burden of disease study. JAMA Oncol. 2017;3(4):524–548.
8. National Cancer Institute: About Cancer: Physical Activity and Cancer. https://www.cancer.gov/about-cancer/causes-prevention/risk/obesity/physical-activity-fact-sheet [Accessed January 6, 2020].
9. Moore S, Lee I, Weiderpass E, et al. Association of leisure-time physical activity with risk of 26 types of cancer in 1.44 million adults. JAMA Intern Med. 2016;176(6):816–825.
10. Breastcancer.org: US Breast Cancer Statistics, 2017. http://www.breastcancer.org/symptoms/understand_bc/statistics [Accessed January 6, 2020].
11. Goncalves A, Dantas Florencio G, et al. Effects of physical activity on breast cancer prevention: a systematic review. J Phys Act Health. 2014;11(2):445–454.
12. Monninkhof E, Elias S, Vlems F, et al. Physical activity and breast cancer: a systematic review. Epidemiology. 2007;18(1):137–157.
13. Steindorf K, Ritte R, Eomois P, et al. Physical activity and risk of breast cancer overall and by hormone receptor status: the European prospective investigation into cancer and nutrition. Int J Cancer. 2013;132(7):1667–1678.
14. Friedenreich C, Woolcott C, McTiernan A, et al. Alberta physical activity and breast cancer prevention trial: sex hormone changes in a year-long exercise intervention among postmenopausal women. J Clin Oncol. 2010;28(9):1458–1466.
15. Mullooly M, Yang H, Falk R, et al. Relationship between crown-like structures and sex-steroid hormones in breast adipose tissue and serum among postmenopausal breast cancer patients. Breast Cancer Res. 2017; 19:8.
16. Wolin K, Yan Y, Colditz G, et al. Physical activity and colon cancer prevention: a meta-analysis. Br J Cancer. 2009;100(4):611–616.

17. Schmid D, Behrens G, Matthews C, et al. Physical activity and risk of colon cancer in diabetic and nondiabetic US adults. Mayo Clin Proc. 2016;91(12):1693–1705.
18. Nilsen T, Romundstad P, Petersen H, et al. Recreational physical activity and cancer risk in subsites of the colon (the Nord-Trondelag Health Study). Cancer Epidem Biomar. 2008;17(1):183–188.
19. Jones L, Peppercorn J, Scott J, et al. Exercise therapy in the management of solid tumors. Curr Treat Option Oncol. 2010;11(0):45–58.
20. Hunter E., Gibson R, Arbesman M, D'Amico M. Systematic review of occupational therapy and adult cancer rehabilitation: Part 1. Impact of physical activity and symptom management interventions. Am J Occup Ther. 2017;71(2):1–11.
21. Brown J, Winters-Stone K, Lee A, et al. Cancer, physical activity, and exercise. Compr Physiol. 2012;2(4):2775–2809.
22. Graydon J, Bubela N, Irvine D, et al. Fatigue-reducing strategies used by patients receiving treatment for cancer. Cancer Nurs. 1995;18(1):23–28.
23. Irwin M, McTiernan A, Manson J, et al. Physical activity and survival in postmenopausal women with breast cancer: results from the women's health initiative. Cancer Prev Res. 2011;4(4):522–529.
24. Friedenreich C, Neilson H, Farris M, et al. Physical activity and cancer outcomes: a precision medicine approach. Clin Cancer Res. 2016;22(19):4766–4775.
25. Hamer J, Warner E. Lifestyle modifications for patients with breast cancer to improve prognosis and optimize overall health. Can Med Assoc J. 2017;189(7):E268–E274.
26. 2018 Physical Activity Guidelines Advisory Committee. 2018 Physical Activity Guidelines Advisory Committee Scientific Report. Washington, DC: U.S. Department of Health and Human Services, 2018.
27. Wolin KY, Schwartz AL, Matthews CE, et al. Implementing the exercise guidelines for cancer survivors. J Support Oncol. 2012;10:171–177.
28. Speck RM, Schmitz KH: Cancer Prevention. http://www.acsm.org/public-information/articles/2016/10/07/cancer-prevention-lifestyle-changes [Accessed January 6, 2020].
29. Rock C, Doyle C, Demark-Wahnefried W, et al. Nutrition and physical activity guidelines for cancer survivors. CA Cancer J Clin. 2012;62(4):243–274.
30. American Institute for Cancer Research: AICR's Guidelines for Cancer Survivors. http://www.aicr.org/patients-survivors/aicrs-guidelines-for-cancer.html [Accessed January 6, 2020].
31. National Comprehensive Cancer Network: Exercising During Cancer Treatment. https://www.nccn.org/patients/resources/life_with_cancer/exercise.aspx [Accessed January 6, 2020].
32. Borch K, Weiderpass E, Braaten T, et al. Physical activity and risk of endometrial cancer in the Norwegian Women and Cancer (NOWAC) study. Int J Cancer. 2017; 140(8):1809–1818.
33. Ekelund U, Ward H, Norat T, et al. Physical activity and all-cause mortality across levels of overall and abdominal adiposity in European men and women: the European prospective investigation into cancer and nutrition study (EPIC). Am J Clin Nutr. 2015;101(3):613–621.
34. WCRF/AICR. Food, Nutrition and the Prevention of Cancer: A Global Perspective Expert Report. 2007.
35. Doyle C, Kushi L, Byers T, et al. 2006 Nutrition, physical activity and cancer survivorship advisory committee; American cancer society. Nutrition and physical activity during and after cancer treatment: an American cancer society guide for informed choices. CA Cancer J Clin. 2006 Nov–Dec;56(6):323–353.
36. Mock V, Atkinson A, Barsevick A, et al. NCCN practice guidelines for cancer-related fatigue. Oncology. 2000;14(11A):151–161.
37. Gerber L. Cancer-related fatigue: persistent, pervasive, and problematic. Phys Med Rehabil Clin N. 2017;28(1):65–88.

38. Haylock P, Hart L. Fatigue in patients receiving localized radiation. Cancer Nurs. 1979;2(6):461–467.
39. Gotte M, Kesting S, Winter C, et al. Experience of barriers and motivations for physical activities and exercise during treatment of pediatric patients with cancer. Pediatr Blood Cancer. 2014;61(9):1632–1637.
40. Yang D, Hausien O, Ageel M, et al. Physical activity levels and barriers to exercise referral among patients with cancer. Patient Educ Couns. 2017;100(7):1402–1407.
41. Ungar N, Wiskemann J, Sieverding M. Physical activity enjoyment and self-efficacy as predictors of cancer patients' physical activity level. Front Psychol. 2016;7:898.
42. Karvinen K, Courneya K, Campbell K, et al. Correlates of exercise motivation and behavior in a population-based sample of endometrial cancer survivors: an application of the theory of planned behavior. Int J Behav Nutr Phy. 2007;4:21.
43. Belanger L, Plotnikoff R, Clark A, et al. A survey of physical activity programming and counseling preferences in young-adult cancer survivors. Cancer Nurs. 2012;35(1):48–54.
44. Komatsu H, Watanuki S, Koyama Y, et al. Nurse counseling for physical activity in patients undergoing esophagectomy. Gastroenterol Nurs. 2016;(3):233–239.
45. Hong Y, Vollmer Dahlke D, Ory M, et al. Designing iCanFit: a mobile-enabled web application to promote physical activity in older cancer survivors. JMIR Res Protoc. 2013;2(1):e12.
46. Robertson M, Tsai E, Lyons E, et al. Mobile health physical activity intervention preferences in cancer survivors: a qualitative study. JMIR Mhealth Uhealth. 2017;5(1):e3.
47. Hellekson K. ACS/ADA/AHA issue core recommendations for preventing cancer, cardiovascular disease, and diabetes. Am Fam Physician. 2005 Feb 15;71(4):806–808.

5 Physical Activity and Diabetes, Prediabetes, and the Metabolic Syndrome

KEY POINTS

- Routine physical activity should be recommended to all individuals who have prediabetes or diabetes (either type 1 or type 2).
- Aerobic activity at a moderate intensity level should be recommended for about 150–175 minutes per week.
- Resistance strength training using major muscle groups should be recommended as two sessions per week with at least a day between the two.
- Physical activity has been routinely shown to lower the risk of diabetes in pre-diabetic individuals and serves as an important component of treatment in individuals with already established diabetes.

5.1   INTRODUCTION

Currently, approximately 9% of the adult population in the United States has type 2 diabetes (T2DM) (1). The associated annual direct medical costs and the lost productivity exceed $245 billion a year (2, 3).

There is a significant role of physical activity across the spectrum of both pre diabetes and diabetes as well as metabolic syndrome. It has been estimated that 150–300 minutes a week of moderate to vigorous physical activity reduces the risk of developing T2DM by 25%–35% (4). These reductions in risk apply to individuals across the weight spectrum from normal weight to overweight or obesity.

In addition to its role of reducing the risk of developing diabetes, regular physical activity can play an important role in the management of diabetes in people who already have the condition. This latter fact is recognized in both the position statement from the American Diabetes Association (ADA) on Physical Activity/ Exercise and Diabetes (5) and the Lifestyle Management Standards for Medical Care in Diabetes 2018 (6).

The purpose of this chapter is to explore the relationship of physical activity across the spectrum of prediabetes, diabetes, and the metabolic syndrome.

Physical activity is generally defined as all movements that increase energy use whereas exercise is typically defined as more planned and structured activity. In addition to lowering the risk or preventing or delaying T2DM development, regular physical activity and exercise also convey health benefits for people with T2DM and type 1 diabetes (T1DM) (5). These health benefits include lower risk of cardiovascular disease, improved cardiovascular fitness, muscle strength, and insulin sensitivity. Since physical activity also results in changes in glucose management, this consideration pertains to individuals with various types of diabetes as they either begin or expand their physical activity program (5, 6).

5.2   TYPES AND CLASSIFICATIONS OF DIABETES AND PREDIABETES

Recommendations for different types of diabetes and precautions related to physical activity may vary considerably depending on its type. There are two primary types of diabetes: type 1 and type 2. In T1DM (5%–10% of cases) there is a cell mediated autoimmune destruction of pancreatic β cells resulting in insulin deficiency (5). In contrast, T2DM (90%–95% of cases) results from progressive loss of insulin secretion and usually insulin resistance (5). Prediabetes is diagnosed when blood glucose levels are above the normal range but not high enough to be classified as diabetes. Individuals in the category of prediabetes, however, have an increased risk of developing T2DM and can prevent or delay its onset with physical activity as well as other lifestyle changes (7, 8).

It should be emphasized that while this chapter will focus on physical activity, other aspects of lifestyle medicine are also crucially important in the reduction of risk of diabetes or management of diabetes. These include medical nutrition therapy and/or weight loss if necessary.

5.3   ADIPOSITY-BASED CHRONIC DISEASE

In addition to the categories of prediabetes and diabetes outlined by the ADA an alternative nomenclature and framework has been suggested by the American Endocrinology Society called adiposity-based chronic disease (ABCD), which refers to the range of chronic disease states resulting from dysglycemia and particularly focused on cardiometabolic risk factors (9). It has been argued that this framework for viewing the spectrum of diseases that result in dysglycemia allows the earliest possible diagnosis of these issues allowing for early preventive strategies including lifestyle interventions such as physical activity, weight loss, and proper nutrition. In addition, it has been argued that the use of ABCD terminology can simplify health messages to patients by combining recommendations for disease prevention with disease treatment.

5.4   TYPES OF EXERCISE AND PHYSICAL ACTIVITY

The types of physical activity and exercise that have been studied in diabetes include aerobic activities that include continuous movement of large muscle groups such as in walking, cycling, jogging. and swimming, where primarily aerobic energy producing systems are utilized (4, 10). Resistance (strength) training involves strength building exercises utilizing free weights, weight machines, or elastic resistance bands or body weight. In addition, flexibility exercises may improve range of motion whereas balance protocols lower the risk of falls and improve gait (11). Activities such as Tai Chi and yoga combine aspects of flexibility, balance, and resistance exercise. Each of these forms of exercises has been utilized in the prevention and treatment of diabetes with variable results (12).

5.4.1   AEROBIC PHYSICAL ACTIVITY

There are multiple benefits from increased aerobic training for reduction of risk and treatment of diabetes. These include improvements in blood vessel reactivity, mitochondrial density, insulin sensitivity, and oxidative enzymes (13). In T1DM, increased cardiorespiratory fitness and decrease in insulin resistance are key responses to increased physical activity. In T1DM, regular physical activity reduces HbA1C, triglycerides, blood pressure, and insulin resistance (13). For all of these reasons the ADA (5), the Canadian Diabetes Canada (14), and the PAGA 2018 Scientific Report all recommend 150–300 minutes of aerobic activity on a weekly basis for both T2DM and T1DM.

5.4.2   RESISTANCE EXERCISE

Resistance exercise has also been demonstrated to have multiple benefits for individuals with diabetes (15). People with diabetes have been found to have lower muscular strength and accelerated decline in functional status (16, 17). Many of these conditions can be ameliorated with resistance training including improvements in muscle mass, body composition, strength, physical function, insulin sensitivity, blood pressure, lipid profiles, and cardiovascular health.

The effect of resistance exercise on glycemic control in T1DM is uncertain (18). Resistance training benefits in T2DM, however, include improvements in glycemic control as well as the abovementioned improvements in body composition (15). For this reason, the ADA, Diabetes Canada, and PAGA 2018 Scientific Report all recommend two sessions of resistance training per week separated by at least one day in T2DM and focusing on all of the major muscle groups.

5.4.3   BENEFITS OF OTHER TYPES OF PHYSICAL ACTIVITY

Flexibility (stretching) and balance exercises are important for older individuals with diabetes. Stretching improves range of motion around joints, but it does not have an impact on glycemic control (11). Balance training can reduce falls and by improving balance and gait even in individuals with diabetes who have peripheral neuropathy (12). There is also some evidence to suggest that Tai Chi classes and yoga may have benefits in improving glycemic control; however, there is less research currently available to support these potential benefits (19).

5.4.4   REDUCING SEDENTARY TIME

Sedentary behavior carries a significant influence on cardiometabolic health. This is particularly important for individuals with diabetes since two-thirds of mortality in individuals with diabetes comes from cardiovascular disease (20, 21). In addition, individuals who either have T2DM or are at risk of developing it have been shown to have poorer glycemic control and increased cluster of metabolic risk such as those found in the metabolic syndrome (22, 23). For all of these reasons, the ADA, Diabetes Canada, and the PAGA 2018 Scientific Report all recommend that individuals with either T2DM or prediabetes should decrease the amount of time spent in sedentary behavior. The recommendation also involves interspersing bouts of light activity with prolonged sitting (22). These recommendations are in addition to, not a replacement for, increased structured exercise or other forms of physical activity.

5.5 PHYSICAL ACTIVITY IN OVERWEIGHT OR OBESE ADULTS WITH T2DM

As already indicated, physical activity is associated with improvements of multiple aspects in individuals with diabetes. The Look AHEAD (Action for Health in Diabetes) trial was the largest randomized trial looking at lifestyle intervention in older adults with T2DM who were overweight or obese (24). The lifestyle intervention was compared with a control that consisted of group support and education. Individuals in the lifestyle intervention were counseled to obtain at least 175 minutes per week of physical activity. They also were targeted to lose at least 7% of weight.

While major cardiovascular events were the same in both groups, the intensive lifestyle intervention group achieved significantly greater sustained improvements in cardiorespiratory fitness, weight loss, blood glucose control, blood pressure, and lipids. In addition, they experienced less sleep apnea and decreased diabetic kidney disease, retinopathy, depression, sexual dysfunction, knee pain, better physical mobility maintenance, and quality of life. These individuals also achieved lower overall health-care costs. The Look AHEAD trial strongly supports the use of physical activity as part of an intensive lifestyle medicine approach to treating overweight or obese individuals with T2DM.

5.6 INSULIN ACTION AND PHYSICAL ACTIVITY

Both regular and acute bouts of physical activity and regular improved insulin action in muscle and liver in individuals with T2DM (25). Aerobic exercise acutely increases blood glucose uptake up to fivefold. After exercise glucose uptake remains elevated for both insulin dependent (approximately 2 hours) and independent (up to 48 hours) actions due to muscle glycogen repletion (26–28).

The goal is to improve insulin action daily. Moderate to high intensity exercise appears to be optimal. In addition, regular exercise training increases oxidative capacity, muscle capillary density, and insulin signaling proteins. Both aerobic and resistance training promote adaptations in skeletal muscle and adipose tissue as well as the liver, which are associated with enhanced insulin action even without weight loss. Some evidence exists that high-intensity interval training may create greater improvements in some of these parameters in individuals with diabetes.

5.7   MANAGEMENT OF FOOD AND INSULIN WITH PHYSICAL ACTIVITY

For individuals with T1DM, blood glucose responses to physical activity are highly variable (29). Aerobic exercise typically decreases blood glucose level in individuals with T1DM. Additional carbohydrate intake or reductions in insulin are typically required for individuals with T1DM who are involved in exercise. Specific recommendations for food intake during physical activity for T1DM are beyond the scope of this chapter. Extensive information, however, is available in this area from the Physical Activity/ Exercise Position Statement of the ADA (5). It should be noted that blood glucose concentration should always be checked prior to exercise in individuals with T1DM.

5.8   PRE-EXERCISE HEALTH SCREENING AND EVALUATION

The ADA has recommended that additional screening beyond usual diabetes care is not necessary to lower the risk of exercise-induced adverse events in asymptotic individuals receiving diabetes care consistent with current ADA guidelines who wish to begin low or moderate intensity physical activity not exceeding the demands of brisk walking or everyday living (5). Individuals who plan to increase their exercise intensity, or who are at high risk, may benefit from a referral to a health-care provider for a checkup and possible exercise stress test prior to starting increased physical activity (30).

The ADA also recommends that adults with diabetes may achieve benefit from working with an exercise physiologist who is knowledgeable about diabetes or certified fitness professional to assist them in formulating a safe and effective exercise prescription (5). The ADA has concluded that careful consideration of multiple factors and clinical judgment will identify the most appropriate physical activities to avoid or limit. These recommendations are slightly less conservative than those promulgated by the American College of Sports Medicine (ACSM), which recommends that currently sedentary individuals with diabetes who want to begin an exercise or increased activity program at any level should obtain medical clearance from a health-care professional prior to beginning (31). The ADA has concluded that the ACSM recommendation is excessively conservative.

5.9   PHYSICAL ACTIVITY IN PREGNANCY WITH DIABETES

Physical activity and exercise in individuals with diabetes have been shown to benefit the majority of women who are pregnant by improving cardiovascular health and general fitness and reducing the risk of complications such as preeclampsia and cesarean delivery (32). Regular physical activity during pregnancy also lowers the risk of developing gestational diabetes mellitus.

The recommendations from the PAGA 2018 Scientific Report (4), ACSM, and ADA (30) include exercise or moderate intensity physical activity of sessions of 20–30 minutes on most days of the week. If gestational diabetes is diagnosed, both aerobic activity and resistance training can improve insulin action and glycemic control (32, 33). There may be an additional benefit of regular physical activity reducing the odds of excessive weight gain during pregnancy.

The ADA recommends, as does the ACSM, that the best time to start a physical activity program is prior to pregnancy but concludes that it is safe to initiate a program of physical activity during pregnancy at moderate intensity levels (30). Of course, symptoms should be carefully monitored by the pregnant woman who is exercising. If a pregnant woman is utilizing insulin, the insulin sensitizing effects of aerobic exercise that have already been discussed in this chapter need to be taken into account particularly during the first trimester.

5.10 MINIMIZING EXERTION OR PHYSICAL ACTIVITY RELATED ADVERSE EVENTS

In individuals with diabetes, as with any physical activity program, it is important take precautions to minimize any potential adverse events. In these individuals, the effect of physical activity on insulin and glucose handling is particularly important. The ADA makes the following recommendations to minimize physical activity adverse events in people with diabetes.

- Make insulin regimen and carbohydrate intake changes to prevent exercise-induced hypoglycemia.
- Reduce the likelihood of nocturnal hypoglycemia following physical activity by reducing basal insulin doses, and including bedtime snacks and/or use of continuous glycose monitoring.
- Hypoglycemia is more common in T1DM than in T2DM but can be mitigated with insulin administration or lower intensity aerobic cool down. If an individual has hyperglycemia or elevated ketones, physical activity should not be conducted.
- Some medications, in addition to insulin, may increase the risk of exercise-related hypoglycemia. Doses of such hypoglycemic medications need to be adjusted based on the amount of physical activity being performed.
- Older adults or anyone who has autonomic neuropathy or cardiovascular complications or pulmonary disease should not exercise outdoors on very hot or humid days to prevent heat-related illnesses.
- Care should be taken to advance exercise training regimens appropriately to minimize the risk of injury.

5.11 PHYSICAL ACTIVITY IN PREDIABETES

Prediabetes is diagnosed when fasting blood glucose levels are above the normal range but not high enough to be classified as diabetes. These are typically between 100 and 120 mg/dL. Individuals with prediabetes are at higher risk of ultimately developing T2DM. A number of studies have now shown, however, that regular physical activity may prevent or delay the onset of diabetes when conducted in conjunction with other lifestyle changes. Two landmark studies demonstrated the power of physical activity as a component of an overall approach to lifestyle interventions to lower this risk of developing diabetes in individuals with prediabetes (7,8).

In the Diabetes Prevention Program (DPP), over 3,000 nondiabetic persons with elevated fasting or post prandial glucose or abnormal glucose tolerance test values entered the intensive lifestyle medicine modification arm of the study with goals of 7% of weight loss and least 150 minutes of physical activity per week. Individuals who participated in this program reduced their risk of developing diabetes by 58% compared to placebo. In addition, the intensive lifestyle intervention was significantly more effective than metformin. The average follow-up in this study was 2.8 years (7).

In the Finnish Diabetes Prevention study (DPS), 522 middle-aged overweight individuals with impaired glucose tolerance were randomized to either a usual care control group or intensive lifestyle medicine intervention (8). The subjects in the intensive lifestyle group received individual dietary counseling from a nutritionist and were offered circuit type resistance training in addition to moderate intensity aerobic physical activity of ≥ 30 minutes a day and weight reduction of ≥ 5%. In follow-up at one and three years, weight reductions were 3.5–4.5 kg in the intervention group. The median amount of moderate intensity physical activity was 160 minutes per week. Individuals in the lifestyle intervention group significantly reduced their risk of developing diabetes.

A recent review of 20 studies showed that individuals who participated in diet and physical activity promotion programs reduced T2DM incidence, body weight, and fasting glucose while improving other cardiometabolic risk factors (34). Programs typically involved 150–175 minutes per week of physical activity, as well as dietary energy restriction and targeted weight loss of 5%–7%. These programs routinely demonstrated reductions of 40%–70% in the risk of developing T2DM in people with impaired glucose tolerance. Thus, the recommendation for including increased amounts of physical activity as part of an overall lifestyle strategy in individuals with prediabetes is a highly effective way of reducing the likelihood of progressing on to diabetes.

5.12 CONCLUSIONS

The ADA, Diabetes Canada, and the PAGA 2018 Scientific Report all recommend increased physical activity to be prescribed to all individuals with diabetes as part of glycemic control and overall health. While specific recommendations vary according to whether individuals are pre-diabetic or diabetic or have T1DM or T2DM, the general recommendation of 150–175 minutes moderate intensity physical activity on a weekly basis is uniform among these three expert recommendations. In addition, all three guidelines recommend two sessions of resistance strength training per week.

There is no serious question that regular physical activity is beneficial at every stage of either prediabetes or diabetes—both for reducing the likelihood of disease progression as an effective adjunct to its treatment.

CLINICAL APPLICATIONS

- Physical activity should be prescribed to all individuals who have either prediabetes (glucose intolerance) or diabetes.
- Aerobic activity for 150–175 minutes per week and two sessions of resistance strength training per week are advocated by the leading professional groups in the management of diabetes.

- All physicians should inquire about the level of physical activity in individuals with prediabetes or diabetes and make appropriate recommendations for enhancing it if that is necessary.
- The amount of time in sedentary pursuits such as sitting should be minimized or broken up with periods of light physical activity in individuals with prediabetes or diabetes.
- Appropriate safety measures involving good regular diabetes care should be employed to minimize adverse events related to physical activity.

REFERENCES

1. Centers for Disease Control and Prevention. National Diabetes Statistics Report 2017. Atlanta, GA: Centers for Disease Control and Prevention, U.S. Department of Health and Human Services, 2017.
2. Centers for Disease Control and Prevention. National Diabetes Statistics Report, 2017: Estimates of Diabetes and Its Burden in the United States. Atlanta, GA: Centers for Disease Control and Prevention, U.S. Department of Health and Human Services; 2017. https://www.cdc.gov/diabetes/pdfs/data/statistics/national-diabetes-statistics-report.pdf. [Accessed December 29, 2019].
3. American Diabetes Association. Economic costs of diabetes in the U.S. in 2012. Diabetes Care. 2013;36(4):1033–1046.
4. Physical Activity Guidelines Advisory Committee. 2018 Physical Activity Guidelines Advisory Committee. Individuals with Chronic Conditions. Washington, DC: U.S. Department of Health and Human Services; 2018.
5. Colberg S, Sigal R, Yardley J, et al. Physical activity/exercise and diabetes: a position statement of the American diabetes association. Diabetes Care. 2016 Nov; 39(11): 2065–2079.
6. American Diabetes Association. Lifestyle management: standards of medical care in diabetes-2018. Diabetes Care. 2018;41(Suppl. 1):S38–S50.
7. The diabetes prevention program (DPP): Description of lifestyle intervention. Diabetes Care. 2002;25:2165–2171.
8. Lindstrom J, Louheranta A, Mannelin M, et al. The Finnish diabetes prevention study (DPS) lifestyle intervention and 3-year results on diet and physical activity. Diabetes Care. 26:3230–3236, 2003.
9. Via M, Mechanick J. Impact of Lifestyle Medicine on Dysglycemia-Based Chronic Disease. In Rippe JM. Lifestyle Medicine (3rd edition). CRC Press (Boca Raton), 2019.
10. 2008 Physical Activity Guidelines for Americans. U.S. Department of Health and Human Services. https://health.gov/paguidelines/2008/pdf/paguide.pdf [Accessed January 13, 2020].
11. Herriott M, Colberg S, Parson H, et al. Effects of 8 weeks of flexibility and resistance training in older adults with type 2 diabetes. Diabetes Care. 2004;27:2988–2989.
12. Morrison S, Colberg S, Mariano M, et al. Balance training reduces falls risk in older individuals with type 2 diabetes. Diabetes Care. 2010;33:748–750.
13. Chimen M, Kennedy A, Nirantharakumar K, et al. What are the health benefits of physical activity in type 1 diabetes mellitus? A literature review. Diabetologia. 2012; 55:542–555.
14. Sigal R, Armstrong M, Bacon S, et al. 2018 Clinical practice guidelines physical activity and diabetes: Diabetes Canada clinical practice guidelines expert committee. Can J Diabetes. 2018;S54–S63.

15. Gordon B, Benson A, Bird S, et al. Resistance training improves metabolic health in type 2 diabetes: a systematic review. Diabetes Res Clin Pract. 2009;83:157–175.
16. Nishitani M, Shimada K, Sunayama S, et al. Impact of diabetes on muscle mass, muscle strength, and exercise tolerance in patients after coronary artery bypass grafting. J Cardiol. 2011;58:173–180.
17. Anton S, Karabetian C, Naugle K, et al. Obesity and diabetes as accelerators of functional decline: can lifestyle interventions maintain functional status in high risk older adults? Exp Gerontol. 2013;48:888–897.
18. Tonoli C, Heyman E, Roelands B, et al. Effects of different types of acute and chronic (training) exercise on glycaemic control in type 1 diabetes mellitus: a meta-analysis. Sports Med. 2012;42:1059–1080.
19. Ahn S, Song R. Effects of tai chi exercise on glucose control, neuropathy scores, balance, and quality of life in patients with type 2 diabetes and neuropathy. J Altern Complement Med. 2012;18:1172–1178.
20. Dempsey P, Owen N, Biddle S, et al. Managing sedentary behavior to reduce the risk of diabetes and cardiovascular disease. Curr Diab Rep. 2014;14:522.
21. Wilmot E, Edwardson C, Achana F, et al. Sedentary time in adults and the association with diabetes, cardiovascular disease and death: systematic review and meta-analysis. Diabetologia. 2012;55:2895–2905.
22. Healy G, Dunstan D, Salmon J, et al. Breaks in sedentary time: beneficial associations with metabolic risk. Diabetes Care. 2008;31:661–666.
23. Fritschi C, Park H, Richardson A, et al. Association between daily time spent in sedentary behavior and duration of hyperglycemia in type 2 diabetes. Biol Res Nurs. 2016:18:160–166.
24. Look AHEAD Research Group, Wing RR, Bolin P, et al. Cardiovascular effects of intensive lifestyle intervention in type 2 diabetes. N Engl J Med. 2013;369:145–154.
25. Roberts C, Hevener A, Barnard R. Metabolic syndrome and insulin resistance: underlying causes and modification by exercise training. Compr Physiol. 2013;3:1–58.
26. Wojtaszewski J, Nielsen J, Richter E. Effect of acute exercise on insulin signaling and action in humans. J Appl Physiol. (1985) 2002;93:384–392.
27. Gillen J, Little J, Punthakee Z, et al. Acute high-intensity interval exercise reduces the postprandial glucose response and prevalence of hyperglycaemia in patients with type 2 diabetes. Diabetes Obes Metab. 2012;14:575–577.
28. Manders R, Van Dijk J, van Loon L. Low intensity exercise reduces the prevalence of hyperglycemia in type 2 diabetes. Med Sci Sports Exerc. 2010;42:219–225.
29. Biankin S, Jenkins A, Campbell L, et al. Target-seeking behavior of plasma glucose with exercise in type 1 diabetes. Diabetes Care. 2003;26:297–301.
30. Colberg S, Sigal R, Fernhall B, et al. American College of sports medicine; American diabetes association. Exercise and type 2 diabetes: the American College of sports medicine and the American diabetes association: joint position statement. Diabetes Care. 2010;33: e147–e167.
31. Riebe D, Franklin B, Thompson P, et al. Updating ACSM's recommendations for exercise preparticipation health screening. Med Sci Sports Exerc. 2015;47:2473–2479.
32. The American College of Obstetricians Gynecologists Committee Obstetric Practice. Physical activity and exercise during pregnancy and the postpartum period. Obstet Gynecol. 2015;126:e135–e142.
33. Colberg S, Castorino K, Jovanovic L. Pre-scribing physical activity to prevent and manage gestational diabetes. World J Diabetes. 2013;4: 256–262.
34. Warburton D, Charlesworth S, Ivey A, et al. A systematic review of the evidence for Canada's physical activity guidelines for adults. Int J Behav Nutr Phys Act. 2010;7:39. doi:10.1186/1479-5868-7-39.

6 Physical Activity in Women's Health

KEY POINTS

- Regular physical activity conveys multiple benefits for women throughout the lifespan.
- Regular physical activity lowers the risk of various chronic diseases including coronary heart disease, diabetes, obesity and weight gain, and certain cancers.
- Regular physical activity is important for brain health and cognition.
- Regular physical activity plays important roles for both pregnancy and post-partum including decreased risk of excessive weight gain and improved fitness and emotional well-being.

6.1 INTRODUCTION

Regular physical activity can play multiple important roles in women's health (1–3). These benefits range from reducing the likelihood of dying from multiple causes to reducing specific risk factors for coronary heart disease (CHD), obesity, diabetes (T2DM), and certain cancers. Cognition affect and other aspects of brain health can also be improved in women with regular physical activity throughout the lifespan.

Regular physical activity can also play important roles both during pregnancy and post-partum as well as menopause (4). In addition, physical activity can play an important role in breast health, bone health, and osteoporosis as well as the preservation of healthy body composition (1–3).

The purpose of the current chapter is to summarize the various ways the physical activity can play important roles in preserving or improving the health of women. Different benefits come from aerobic exercise compared to resistance training, however, both are important.

Multiple organizations including the American Heart Association (AHA) (5), Physical Activity Guidelines for Americans 2008 (6) and 2018 (3), and the American College of Sports Medicine (ACSM) (7) have all issued guidelines and recommendations for regular exercise. Typically these guidelines involve 30 minutes of moderate intensity physical activity on most days or perhaps vigorous intensity physical activity of at least 25 minutes two or three days a week.

Unfortunately, only approximately 28% of women exercise enough to meet these basic guidelines and 41% engage in no physical activity at all (8). Aerobic activity has been the focus of most research on health benefits for women. Resistance exercise, however, may also confer health benefits particularly in the area of bone density and musculoskeletal function. Yet only 17.5% of women engage in strength training at least twice a week which is recommended by the current guidelines (9–11).

While most of the recommendations involve 30 minutes of moderate intensity physical activity on most days and two sessions of resistance strength training per week, even much smaller levels of regular physical activity can substantially reduce the risk of various chronic illnesses. Moreover, there is a dose/response relationship such that individuals who exercise at higher levels than the current recommendations may derive additional benefits (3). All these issues will also be explored in this chapter.

While this chapter will focus on largely on aerobic physical activity, other risk factors that have to do with lifestyle decisions may also significantly impact on the likelihood of developing various chronic diseases including CHD and Type 2 Diabetes (T2DM). For example, the Nurses' Health Trial demonstrated that 84% of all CHD and 91% of diabetes could be eliminated if women followed five simple practices including regular physical activity (30 minutes on most days), maintain a proper healthy weight (BMI <25 kg/m^2), follow sound nutritional practices (e.g. more fruits and vegetables, whole grains and several fish meals a week), do not smoke cigarettes, and consume only moderate amounts of alcohol (1 alcohol beverage per day) (2).

6.2   ALL-CAUSE MORTALITY

Multiple prospective and cohort studies show inverse associations between physical activity and all-cause mortality. The Physical Guidelines for Americans 2008 estimated a 30% decrease in risk of all-cause mortality when comparing the least to most active individuals (6). Further risk decreases were noted in the 2018 Physical Activity Guidelines for Americans Scientific Report (3). Even individuals who exercised only 30 minutes per week achieved a 20% decrease in risk of all-cause mortality, while individuals who exercised 1.5 hours per week had a further 30% reduction in all-cause mortality. Recent evidence utilizing accelerometers showed that there was a reduction in risk factors for heart disease of 60–70% in women when comparing the highest to the lowest levels of physical activity (12).

In a meta-analysis of 22 large cohort studies involving 643,000 women and 335,000 men those who performed 2.5 hours per week of moderate intensity physical activity (equivalent of 30 minutes a day, 5 days a week) experienced a 19% reduction in all-cause mortality, while those who performed 30 minutes of moderate activity on a daily basis reduced their mortality risk by 24% (13).

According to the National Institute of Health (NIH), American Association of Retired Persons (AARP) Diet and Health Study which involved 253,000 women, those who engaged in moderate intensity physical activity 3 hours or greater experienced a 27% decrease in risk of mortality compared to no physical activity (14). Those who engaged in vigorous activity for 20 minutes greater than 3 times a week achieved a 32% reduction in risk (15).

In addition, a number of studies have shown that time spent in sedentary living represents an independent risk factor for all-cause mortality. The American Cancer Society's Cancer Prevention Study II (CPS-II) showed that individuals who were involved in sitting greater than six hours per day experienced a 37% increase in mortality (16). Those who were involved in sedentary occupations, yet managed to maintain recommended levels of physical activity were able to substantially ameliorate this risk (17).

6.3 PHYSICAL ACTIVITY AND CORONARY HEART DISEASE (CHD)

Physical activity plays a substantial role in reducing the risk of CHD in women (16). This is particularly important since CHD is the leading cause of death in women by age 65. Since women tend to get serious manifestations of heart disease such as myocardial infarction (MI) and sudden cardiac death at a later age than men, women who have developed CHD have a significantly worse prognosis than men. Unfortunately, in a national survey of physician awareness of CHD prevention guidelines, less than one in five physicians knew that more women than men die each year because of CHD (1).

Multiple studies have shown that 30 minutes per day of moderate intensity physical activity substantially lowers the risk of CHD in women. In the Women's Health Initiative Observational Study (18), walking briskly for at least 2.4 hours per week (approximately 30 minutes five times per week) was associated with a 30% reduction in cardiovascular events over a 3.2 year follow up. In an 8 year follow up study of 72,000 healthy middle aged female nurses three hours of brisk walking or 1.5 hours of vigorous exercise per week resulted in a 30–40% lower risk of MI compared to sedentary individuals (19). Other studies have shown similar benefits.

It used to be thought that physical activity needed to be at least ten minutes in duration per session to yield benefits. The most recent data, however, summarized in the PAGA 2018 Scientific Report showed that any level of increased physical activity will result in reduced risk of CHD (20). In addition to aerobic physical activity, women who train with weights greater than 30 minutes per week are 23% less likely to develop CHD over an 8 year follow up, yet only 17.5% women engage in strength training at this level (21).

6.4 PHYSICAL ACTIVITY AND TYPE 2 DIABETES

Many studies have demonstrated that regular physical activity lowers the risk of diabetes in women. In the Women's Health Study participants who reported walking 2–3 hours per week were 34% less likely to develop T2DM over a 7 year follow-up compared to those who reported not walking (22). In a study of 4,369 middle aged Finnish women and men, followed for 9.4 years, individuals who walked or cycled to work for at least 30 minutes per day experienced a 36% reduction in the risk of T2DM compared to peers who did not engage in these activities (23).

It should be noted that physical inactivity and obesity independently contribute to the development of both CHD and T2DM in initially healthy women. Furthermore, regular physical activity with or without concomitant weight loss can prevent or postpone diabetes onset as reported in a variety of intervention studies.

It is thought that regular physical activity slows the initiation and progression of diabetes through a variety of favorable effects including lower body weight, increased insulin sensitivity, improved glycemic control, lower blood pressure, improved lipid profile, enhanced endothelial function, improved hemostasis, and more effective inflammatory defense systems (24). One randomized controlled study showed that a combination of aerobic and resistance exercise lowered the risk of diabetes more than either modality alone (24). Both the Diabetes Prevention Program (DPP) (25) and the Finnish Diabetes Study (23) showed significant decreases in the likelihood of developing diabetes in individuals with impaired fasting glucose who were involved in physical activity 150 minutes per week and achieved a 5–7% loss of body weight.

More detail about the relationship between physical activity and diabetes in both men and women may be found in Chapter 5.

6.5   WEIGHT CONTROL

The United States and much of the developed world are in the midst of pandemics of overweight and obesity (26). Regular physical activity is an important adjunct to weight loss programs and very important to lower the risk of weight gain in healthy weight women. While physical activity alone yields only modest benefit in terms of initial weight loss (on the order of 2–3%), regular physical activity is very important for the long-term maintenance of weight loss (27). Numerous studies have documented that both caloric restriction and physical activity play important roles in long-term maintenance of weight loss. Despite these data, only 20% of adults in the United States who are attempting to lose weight report using a combination of energy restriction and engaging in ≥150 minutes of moderate intensity physical activity per week (28). More details concerning the link between physical activity and reducing the risk of weight gain and obesity may be found in Chapter 10.

6.6   CANCER

Physical activity has been shown to significantly reduce the risk of multiple cancers in women. As a result of this, both the American Cancer Society and the PAGA 2018 Scientific Report (29) recommend 30 minutes of moderate to vigorous intensity physical activity on 5 or more days per week.

Both the World Cancer Research Fund and the American Institute of Cancer Research have concurred with these recommendations and noted that regular physical activity has been associated with significant reductions in the prevalence and risk of 13 different cancers including breast, endometrial, and colon cancer (30) in women. The mechanism for why regular physical activity lowers the risk of various cancers is not completely known. Moreover, since there are a variety of different etiologies for cancer it is likely that there are multiple different mechanisms.

6.6.1   Breast Cancer

Several systematic reviews of cohort and case studies have documented an average decrease of 25% the risk of breast cancer when comparing the most physically active to the most least physically active women (31). In the Nurses' Health Study women who engaged in physical activity at approximately one hour per day of brisk walking were 15% less likely to develop breast cancer than those who were sedentary (1). There also appears to be a dose/response relationship with higher levels of physical activity further reducing the risk of breast cancer. Moreover, physical activity as part of the comprehensive treatment for breast cancer has also resulted in survival benefits.

6.6.2   COLON CANCER

A number of studies have shown that there is an inverse relationship between physical activity and risk of colon cancer in both men and women. The risk reduction varies from 20–30% when comparing the most active to the least active women depending on the specific parameters studied (32). Among the 79,000 participants in the Nurses' Health Study who were followed for up to 16 years, there was a 23% risk reduction comparing the most active to the least active women (33). The most active women were involved in the equivalent of brisk walking for approximately 5–6 hours per week. A faster walking pace was also associated with reduced risk. Women, who participated in moderate or vigorous physical activity other than walking, showed a 44% lower risk of colon cancer if they exercised more than 4 hours per week.

6.6.3   ENDOMETRIAL CANCER

A meta-analysis of 11 prospective cohort studies found a significant inverse relationship between physical activity and endometrial cancer (34). Reduction in risk was approximately 27% even when adjusting for obesity and BMI. There may be a dose/response relationship involved with physical activity and reduction risk of endometrial cancer. In the NIH AARP Diet and Health Study, women who were followed for an average of 7 years showed a decreased risk of endometrial cancer for vigorous physical activity but not light or moderate physical activity (35).

6.6.4   OVARIAN CANCER

It remains unclear whether physical activity plays a role in the prevention of ovarian cancer. One meta-analysis showed that there was a 20% reduced risk for the most active versus the least active women (36). Other studies have not yielded a protective effect of physical activity in ovarian cancer.

6.6.5   LUNG CANCER

A systematic review of 20 cohort and 7 case control studies of physical activity and lung cancer risk concluded that physical activity was associated with a risk reduction of 20–30% in women and 20–50% (37) in men. Most studies have not accounted for the effect of cigarette smoking, but not all studies. Thus, there is the potential for some confusion in these data.

6.6.6   OTHER CANCERS

An expanded array of cancers where physical activity has been shown to lower the risk was documented in the Physical Activity Guidelines for Americans 2018 Scientific Report. More detail concerning these relationships is found in Chapter 4.

6.7   BREAST HEALTH

In addition to lowering the risk of breast cancer, regular physical activity improves mood, increases self-esteem and creates a positive body image (38). Regular exercise improves muscle tone, strength, and endurance and has protective effect of decreasing risk of CHD and T2DM. Regular exercise can also lower body weight which, in turn, reduces the risk of breast cancer due to overweight and obesity.

6.8   BRAIN HEALTH/COGNITIVE FUNCTION

Physical activity has been shown to be associated with multiple aspects of cognitive function and brain health throughout the lifespan in women (39–41). In 2009, a meta-analysis of 16 prospective studies reported that individuals in the highest activity category experienced a 28% reduction in the risk of dementia and a 45% reduction in the risk of Alzheimer's disease compared to individuals in the lowest activity category (42). In addition, regular physical activity is associated with improved cognition including executive function (43), and improved affect including lower risk of both depression and anxiety. All of these factors are, of course, are important given the increasing age of the population in the United States and the rest of the developed world. Much more detail concerning the effects of regular physical activity on brain health and cognition may be found in Chapter 11.

6.9   PREGNANCY AND POST-PARTUM

Physical activity yields multiple benefits during pregnancy and post-partum. For this reason, both the American College of Obstetrics and Gynecology (ACOG) (4) and the PAGA 2018 Scientific Report recommend regular physical activity for women who are pregnant (3).

Both ACOG (4) and the PAGA 2018 (3) recommend at least 150 minutes per week of moderate intensity aerobic activity spread throughout the week in periods of approximately 30 minutes per session. The specific recommendations for moderate intensity physical activity include such activities as walking, swimming, or low impact aerobics. Regular moderate intensity exercise during pregnancy lowers the risk of excessive weight gain during pregnancy and also lowers the risk of gestational diabetes.

The ACOG Guidelines indicate that physical activities that should be avoided include contact sports, or activities with high risk of falling (e.g., downhill snow skiing, water skiing, surfing, off road cycling, gymnastics, and horseback riding) as well as scuba diving, sky diving, and "hot yoga" or "hot Pilates."

Pregnant individuals who are contemplating vigorous exercise such as racquet sports or strength training should consult their health care provider although women who have been involved in these activities regularly before pregnancy should be able to continue them safely. An additional benefit of physical activity during pregnancy includes the ability to maintain physical fitness. Women should utilize ratings of perceived exertion rather than heart rate to gauge intensity of exercise and should not exceed perceived exertion of 13–14 on the 6–20 Borg Scale of Perceived Exertion. This corresponds to exercise that is "somewhat hard."

Both the PAGA 2008 (6) and PAGA 2018 Scientific Report (3) found limited evidence to suggest that regular physical activity reduced the risk of anxiety and depression during pregnancy (3). The Committee also found that there was strong evidence of an inverse relationship between physical activity and reduced symptoms of depression during post-partum.

6.10   MENOPAUSE

Regular physical activity may be an important component of health including both physical and psychological well-being during menopause. Individuals in menopause have been reported to have more energy and a better sense of well-being if they are engaged in regular physical activity (44). In addition, aerobic exercise is well known to produce multiple benefits for reducing the risk of developing CVD, T2DM, weight gain, and obesity.

Data on physical activity for vasomotor symptoms during menopause are limited although a sense of well-being and control over various aspects of physiologic function during menopause may be important benefits from regular physical activity. In addition, regular physical activity may ameliorate depressive symptoms during menopause although data in this area is inconclusive.

6.11   BONE HEALTH/OSTEOPOROSIS

A number of randomized controlled trials (RCTs) have assessed the relationship between physical activity and bone mineral density (BMD) in women. In 2011, a meta-analysis of 43 such trials on post-menopausal women which utilized a variety of exercise types showed slower bone loss at the spine by 3.2% and at the hip by 1% (45). Both of these are highly significant. However, these trials lasted less than 12 months so it cannot be determined at this point whether or not regular physical activity actually resulted in fewer fractures of the hip or compression fractures of the spine.

Osteoporosis is a significant public health problem particularly in women who are in menopause which appears to be related to a decrease in estrogen level. Physical activity may reduce the risk of osteoporotic fractures by increasing bone strength (particularly weight bearing aerobic and strength training exercise) and also preventing falls (resistance, balance, and flexibility exercise).

Trials exploring physical activity in relation to fracture risk have largely focused on hip fracture since this is a significant medical issue for many older individuals and can be monitored by exploring medical records. In 2008, a meta-analysis of 13 prospective trials showed that moderate to vigorous physical activity was associated with a hip fracture risk reduction of 38% in women (46). In the Nurses' Health Study with a follow up of 12 years, each increase of one hour per week of walking at an average pace was associated with a 6% reduction in risk of hip fracture. Women who reported walking more than 4 hours per week had a 41% lower risk of hip fracture compared to individuals who walked less than one hour per week (45).

With regard to risk of vertebral fracture, moderate to vigorous physical activity (greater than 2 hours per day) reduced the risk for radiographically assessed vertebral fracture by 33% in women compared with no activity (47).

6.12   PHYSICAL ACTIVITY AND BODY COMPOSITION

Physical activity carries multiple benefits for improving various aspects of body composition. In particular, studies have shown a variety of improvements in lean muscle and reduction of adiposity (48). Muscular strength through regular physical activity also enhances physical independence and the ability to perform activities of daily living and enjoy recreational pursuits. Regular physical activity (particularly resistance strength training) also helps prevent the age-related loss of muscle (sarcopenia) and frailty. Frailty is associated with early mortality.

In a 12 year study of 14,713 individuals, 54% of whom were women, individuals who were relatively fit had a lower mortality and fewer fractures than unfit people. Physical activity also helps preserve bone health and is an important component of successful long-term weight management. In particular, weight loss studies which have utilized energy restriction alone rather than a combination of energy restriction and physical activity have shown that 25–33% of weight loss during periods of short-term weight loss is lean muscle mass which decreases strength and lowers metabolic rate. The most effective physical activity regimen for maintaining optimal body weight in women involves the combination of regular physical activity, strength training, and increased activities of daily living.

6.13   SPORTS AND PHYSICAL ACTIVITY FOR GIRLS AND WOMEN

As outlined in multiple chapters in this book, regular physical activity is associated with improvements in health across the lifespan for both men and women. Participation in sports and physical activity during adolescence is strongly associated with adult physical activity levels (49). In addition, as already indicated, the risk of developing various chronic diseases such as CHD, T2DM, and dementia is reduced by regular physical activity in women.

The 2018 Physical Activity Guidelines for Americans Scientific Report recommended that girls (and boys) age 6–17 years should participate in 60 minutes or more of moderate to vigorous physical activity every day. Physical activity in girls lowers the risk of developing chronic disease and also improves self-esteem and cognition.

Physical activity in young adolescent girls (49) should include a variety of age appropriate activities including aerobic activities, muscle strengthening, and bone strengthening. Despite these recommendations, the 2016 US Report Card on Physical Activity in Children and Youth found that only 21.6% of 6–19 years old children and adolescents in the United States attained 60 or more minutes of moderate aerobic physical activity on at least five days per week. As children age, physical activity generally declines particularly amongst girls. Slightly more than 70% of elementary school aged girls achieve 60 minutes of moderate or vigorous activity on 7 days a week but that number declines to 22.5% for high school females (49).

Oftentimes, physical activity programs are school-based. Unfortunately, school-based programs have declined in number significantly over the past 30 years. In 1991, 42% of high school students had physical education five days per week but this had declined to 29% by 2015. A large body of literature has shown that students who are physically active perform better in school, achieve better grades, are more likely to attend school, improve cognitive performance and classroom behaviors. Thus, physical activity for women and girls is very important. One of the great ways to enhance physical activity for both women and girls is to encourage active participation not only in leisure time physical activity, but also in various sports.

6.14   RISKS OF PHYSICAL ACTIVITY

Despite its many benefits, physical activity does carry certain risks. These include musculoskeletal injuries, rare acute cardiac events, and menstrual dysfunction. Musculoskeletal injuries vary by activity type. Low impact activities such as walking, swimming, cycling, and gardening are associated with the fewest risks (3, 6).

Research has shown that when individuals increase their usual amount of physical activity rapidly, the risk of injury is related to the size of the increase. For this reason, gradual, modest increases in physical activity are appropriate to reduce injury risk. Physical exertion can also trigger acute cardiac events. This appears true for both men and women. The increase in incidence of acute cardiac events during physical activity, however, is very low; 2–3 events per 10,000 person years for heart attacks and one event per 10,000 person years for sudden cardiac death (50). Habitual physical activity significantly lowers the association between episodic physical activity and adverse cardiac events.

There is also an adverse potential particularly in adolescent girls of menstrual dysfunction which has focused largely on competitive athletes who are performing high levels of exercise and training. ACSM coined the term "female athlete triad" to describe a constellation of disordered eating, amenorrhea, and osteoporosis which may occur in some competitive athletes (49). Women engaged in sports which emphasize lean body types such as gymnastics, ballet, figure skating, and long distance running are particularly susceptible to this condition. This suggests that physical activity is not the main culprit of this condition and energy balance but not expenditure plays the most significant role.

6.15   SUMMARY/CONCLUSIONS

Regular physical activity results in multiple benefits for women throughout the lifespan. Regular physical activity lowers the risk of various chronic diseases such as CHD, T2DM, obesity, and some cancers. Regular physical activity has been demonstrated in numerous studies to result in decreased risk of all-cause mortality. In addition, regular physical activity plays a significant role in overall breast health, brain health and cognition, and bone health. Furthermore, regular physical activity yields multiple benefits in pregnancy and post-partum as well as in menopause. Thus, there are numerous important related benefits of regular physical activity for women throughout the lifespan.

CLINICAL APPLICATIONS

- Regular physical activity should be encouraged in girls and women throughout the lifespan
- All clinicians should assess the level of physical activity and, if needed, recommend increases

- Physical activity prescription in women should involve an understanding of current fitness levels and should involve activities with low injury potential
- Regular physical activity has been shown to yield multiple benefits in pregnancy and post-partum
- Regular physical activity also conveys multiple benefits in menopause including improvements in bone health. Thus, levels of physical activity should be assessed and recommended in all women in this age group.

REFERENCES

1. Bassuk S, Manson J. Physical activity and health in women. In Rippe, JM. Lifestyle Medicine (2nd edition). CRC Press (Boca Raton, FL), 2013.
2. Bassuk S, Manson J. Lifestyle and risk of cardiovascular disease and type 2 diabetes in women: a review of the epidemiologic evidence. Amer J Lifestyle Med. 2018;2:191–213.
3. Physical Activity Guidelines Advisory Committee. 2018 Physical Activity Guidelines Advisory Committee. 2018 Physical Activity Guidelines Advisory Committee Scientific Report. Women Who Are Pregnant or Postpartum. Washington, DC: U.S. Department of Health and Human Services.
4. The American College of Obstetricians and Gynecologists. https://www.acog.org/About-ACOG/ACOG-Departments/Deliveries-Before-39-Weeks/ACOG-Clinical-Guidelines?IsMobileSet=false [Accessed: January 9, 2020].
5. American Heart Association. https://www.heart.org/en/news/category-womens-health [Accessed: January 9, 2020].
6. U.S. Department of Health and Human Services. 2008 Physical Activity Guidelines for Americans. https://health.gov/paguidelines/2008/ [Accessed: January 8, 2020].
7. American College of Sports Medicine. 2018 Guidelines for Exercise Testing and Prescription (10th edition). Wolters Kluwer (Philadelphia, PA), 2018.
8. Barnes PM. Physical Activity among Adults: United States, 2000 and 2005. Hyattsville, MD: U.S. Department of Health and Human Services, Centers for Disease Control; 2007. Available at http://www.cdc.gov/nchs/data/hestat/physicalactivity/physicalactivity.htm [Accessed: January 9, 2020].
9. U.S. Department of Health and Human Services. 2008 Physical Activity Guidelines for Americans. ODPHP Publication No. U0336, October 2008. Available at http://www.health.gov/paguidelines/guidelines/default.aspx [Accessed: January 9, 2020].
10. Williams MA, Haskell WL, Ades PA et al. Resistance exercise in individuals with and without cardiovascular disease: 2007 update: a scientific statement from the American heart association council on clinical cardiology and council on nutrition, physical activity, and metabolism. Circulation. 2007;116:572–584,.
11. Carey V, Walters E, Colditz G, et al. Body fat distribution and risk of Non-insulin dependent diabetes mellitus in women: the Nurses' health study. Am J Epidemiol. 1997;145(7):614–619.
12. Lee I, Shiroma E, Evenson K, et al. Accelerometer-measured physical activity and sedentary behavior in relation to all-cause mortality: the women's health study. Circulation. 2018;137:203–205.
13. Woodcock J, Franco O, Orsini N, et al. Non-vigorous physical activity and all-cause mortality: systematic review and meta-analysis of cohort studies. Int J Epidemiol. 2011;40:121–138.
14. Hamer M, Chida Y. Walking and primary prevention: a meta-analysis of prospective cohort studies. Br J Sports Med. 2008;42:238–243.
15. Leitzmann MF, Park Y, Blair A et al. Physical activity recommendations and decreased risk of mortality. Arch Intern Med. 2007;167:2453–2460.

16. Patel AV, Bernstein L, Deka A et al. Leisure time spent sitting in relation to total mortality in a prospective cohort of US adults. Am J Epidemiol. 2010;172:419–429.
17. 2018 Physical Activity Guidelines Advisory Committee. Physical Activity Guidelines Advisory Committee Scientific Report. Washington, DC: U.S. Department of Health and Human Services, 2018. Sedentary Behavior Part F. Chapter 2.
18. Manson JE, Greenland P, LaCroix AZ et al. Walking compared with vigorous exercise for the prevention of cardiovascular events in women. N Engl J Med. 2002;347:716–725.
19. Manson JE, Hu FB, Rich-Edwards JW et al. A prospective study of walking as compared with vigorous exercise in the prevention of coronary heart disease in women. N Engl J Med. 1999;341:650–658.
20. Physical Activity Guidelines Advisory Committee. 2018 Physical Activity Guidelines Advisory Committee Scientific Report. Washington DC: US Department of Health and Human Services; 2018.
21. Tanasescu M, Leitzmann MF, Rimm EB, Willett WC, et al. Stampfer MJ, Hu FB. Exercise type and intensity in relation to coronary heart disease in men. JAMA. 2002;288:1994–2000.
22. Weinstein AR, Sesso HD, Lee IM et al. Relationship of physical activity vs. Body mass index with type 2 diabetes in women. JAMA. 2004;292:1188–1194.
23. Tuomilehto J, Lindstrom J, Eriksson JG et al. Prevention of type 2 diabetes mellitus by changes in lifestyle among subjects with impaired glucose tolerance. N Engl J Med. 2001; 344:1343–1350.
24. Colberg S, Sigal R, Yardley J, et al. Physical activity/exercise and diabetes: a position statement of the American diabetes association. Diabetes Care. 2016;39:2065–2079.
25. Knowler WC, Barrett-Connor E, Fowler SE, et al. Diabetes prevention program research group. Reduction in the incidence of type 2 diabetes with lifestyle intervention or metformin. N Engl J Med. 2002;346:393–403.
26. Centers for Disease Control and Prevention. 2018. Adult Obesity Facts. https://www.cdc.gov/obesity/data/adult.html [Accessed: January 10, 2020].
27. The National Weight Control Registry. http://www.nwcr.ws/ [Accessed January 10, 2020].
28. Rippe JM. Lifestyle medicine: the health promoting power of daily habits and practices. Am J Lifestyle Med. 2018;12:499–512.
29. Physical Activity Guidelines Advisory Committee. 2018 Physical Activity Guidelines Advisory Committee Scientific Report. Washington, DC: U.S. Department of Health and Human Services, 2018. Cancer Prevention Part F. Chapter 4. 2018.
30. World Cancer Research Fund and the American Institute for Cancer Research. Food, Nutrition, Physical Activity, and the Prevention of Cancer: A Global Perspective. Washington, DC: American Institute for Cancer Research. 2007.
31. Lynch BM, Neilson HK, Friedenreich CM. Physical activity and breast cancer prevention. In: Courneya KS, Friedenreich CM, eds. Physical Activity and Cancer, Springer-Verlag (Berlin, Germany), 2011.
32. Wolin KY, Yan Y, Colditz GA, et al. Physical activity and colon cancer prevention: a meta-analysis. Br J Cancer. 2009;100:611–616.
33. Wolin KY, Lee IM, Colditz GA, et al. Leisure-time physical activity patterns and risk of colon cancer in women. Int J Cancer. 2007;121:2776–2781.
34. Moore SC, Gierach GL, Schatzkin A, et al. Physical activity, sedentary behaviours, and the prevention of endometrial cancer. Br J Cancer. 2010;103:933–938.
35. Gierach GL, Chang SC, Brinton LA et al. Physical activity, sedentary behavior, and endometrial cancer risk in the NIH-AARP diet and health study. Int J Cancer. 2009; 124:2139–2147.
36. Olsen CM, Bain CJ, Jordan SJ et al. Recreational physical activity and epithelial ovarian cancer: a case–control study, systematic review, and meta-analysis. Cancer Epidemiol Biomarkers Prev. 2007;16:2321–2330.

37. Emaus A, Thune I. Physical activity and lung cancer prevention. In: Courneya KS, Friedenreich CM, eds. Physical Activity and Cancer, 101–133.Springer-Verlag (Berlin, Germany), 2011.

38. Dupree B. Breast health: Lifestyle modification. In Rippe, JM. Lifestyle Medicine (2nd edition), 287–298. CRC Press (Boca Raton, FL), 2013.

39. Kramer AF, Erickson KI, Colcombe SJ. Exercise, cognition, and the aging brain. J Appl Physiol. 2006;101:1237–1242.

40. Weuve J, Kang JH, Manson JE, et al. Physical activity, including walking, and cognitive function in older women. JAMA. 2004;292:1454–1461.

41. Yaffe K, Barnes D, Nevitt M, et al. A prospective study of physical activity and cognitive decline in elderly women: women who walk. Arch Intern Med. 2001;161:1703–1708.

42. Hamer M, Chida Y. Physical activity and risk of neurodegenerative disease: a systematic review of prospective evidence. Psychol Med. 2009;39:3–11.

43. Colcombe S, Kramer AF. Fitness effects on the cognitive function of older adults: a meta-analytic study. Psychol Sci. 2003;14:125–130.

44. Gass M. Menopause. In Rippe, JM. Lifestyle Medicine (2nd edition), 281–286. CRC Press (Boca Raton, FL), 2013.

45. Howe TE, Shea B, Dawson LJ et al. Exercise for preventing and treating osteoporosis in postmenopausal women. Cochrane Database Syst Rev. CD000333. 2011.

46. Feskanich D, Willett W, Colditz G. Walking and leisure-time activity and risk of hip fracture in postmenopausal women. JAMA. 2002;288:2300–2306.

47. Gregg EW, Cauley JA, Seeley DG, et al. Physical activity and osteoporotic fracture risk in older women. Study of osteoporotic fractures research group. Ann Intern Med. 1998;129:81–88.

48. Peeke PM. Women's body composition and lifestyle. In Rippe, JM. Lifestyle Medicine (2nd edition), 331–341. CRC Press (Boca Raton, FL), 2013.

49. Joy L, Sports and physical activity for women and girls. The role of rehabilitation in injury management. In Rippe, JM. Lifestyle Medicine (2nd edition). CRC Press (Boca Raton, FL), 2013.

50. Dahabreh IJ, Paulus JK. Association of episodic physical and sexual activity with triggering of acute cardiac events: systematic review and meta-analysis. JAMA. 2011;305:1225–1233.

7 Physical Activity and Youth

KEY POINTS

- Increased physical activity results in multiple health and fitness benefits for children and adolescents between the agteses of 3 and 17.
- Multiple guidelines recommend 60 minutes of moderate to vigorous physical activity (MVPA) on a daily basis and three sessions of musculoskeletal training on a weekly basis for this group.
- Unfortunately, 80% of children do not achieve these recommended levels.
- Increased physical activity has been demonstrated to be strongly associated with cardiometabolic health, cardiovascular fitness, weight control, bone health, and cognitive health in children and adolescents.
- Conversely, sedentary behavior has been associated with increased risk factors for chronic disease in children.
- Since physical activity in children is likely to track into adulthood, it is even more imperative that efforts be made by clinicians to help children and families increase their levels of physical activity.

7.1 INTRODUCTION

It is well known that many of the roots of chronic diseases that become manifest in adults have their roots in childhood (1). Thus, it is very important to explore how lifestyle issues, in general, and physical activity, in particular, can play a role in the health and wellbeing of children as well as reducing their risk of chronic disease.

Numerous studies have shown that regular physical activity can have beneficial effects on reducing multiple risk factors for cardiovascular disease (CVD) including lipids, blood pressure and blood glucose (2–4). In addition, regular physical activity can play an important role in body composition, aerobic fitness, muscular strength, movement skills, and bone health (4). An emerging literature has shown that regular physical activity can also improve academic performance and feelings of wellbeing (5). Participating in regular physical activity also tracks well into adulthood, thus, carrying additional benefits.

Physical inactivity is a global health issue and also has its roots in childhood. The current Physical Activity Guidelines from multiple sources in the United States (1) and around the world call for children and youth to participate in at least 60 minutes of moderate or vigorous physical activity on a daily basis (6–9). In addition, guidelines recommend muscle and bone strengthening activities performed at least three days per week. These guidelines are supported by the Physical Activity Guidelines for Americans 2018 Scientific Report (PAGA 2018) as well as organizations such as the American Heart Association (AHA) (10) and the American College of Sports Medicine (ACSM) (4).

Unfortunately, 80% of adolescents do not achieve the recommended Guidelines for Moderate to Vigorous Physical Activity (MVPA) (11). According to the 2016 U.S. Report Card on Physical Activity in Children and Youth, the overall grade for physical activity performance levels is a D– and for active transportation a resounding "F." In addition, sedentary behaviors achieve a D– and school programs are not doing much better, with a rating of D+.

According to the Physical Activity Guidelines Advisory Committee Report of 2008 (12), strong evidence confirmed that children and adolescents between the ages of 6 and 17 receive multiple health benefits including cardiorespiratory and muscular fitness, bone health, and maintenance of a healthy weight status by participating in regular physical activity. The 2018 PAGA Scientific Report extended these findings to children between the ages of 3 and 6, since additional information became available in the decade between 2008 and 2018 relating to this younger population. In particular, the PAGA 2018 concluded that in children of age 3–6, increased amounts of physical activity were associated with improved bone health and reduction in risk of excessive increases in body weight and adiposity (13–16). These findings are particularly important since approximately 13 million children representing more than 4% of the US population are younger than age 6.

This chapter will largely focus on the health and fitness benefits of regular physical activity in children age 6–17, although, as already indicated, somewhat similar information is available for children between the ages 3 and 6.

7.2   PHYSICAL ACTIVITY AND CARDIOMETABOLIC HEALTH

An inactive lifestyle is associated with the development of atherosclerotic CVD, type 2 diabetes (T2DM), and many other diseases (17–20). An inactive lifestyle has also been linked to a number of biological risk factors for these diseases such as hypertension, hyperlipidemia, and insulin resistance (17–20). While these diseases are not usually manifested in children, the precursors of atherosclerosis such as fatty streaks in the arteries can be seen in children and the degree of these atherosclerotic precursors is related to the level of CVD risk factors in adults. In addition, T2DM, which has typically been associated with adults, has become increasingly common in children.

While no studies have specifically examined the progression of atherosclerosis from childhood into clinical manifestations in adults, associations have been found between physical inactivity and arterial stiffness and wall thickness (21–22). The PAGA 2018 Scientific Report identifies one systematic review and several meta-analyses that explore the association between physical activity and cardiometabolic health in children and adolescents. The meta-analyses routinely showed that physical activity resulted in significant lowering of plasma triglycerides. Most of these meta-analyses also showed that physical activity lowered plasma insulin levels (23). While the results for high-density lipoprotein cholesterol and blood pressure were not very strong (24–25), there was some suggestion that physical activity resulted in the benefit of improvements in both of these. It should also be noted that physical activity in childhood may influence physical activity levels in adulthood.

With all of these findings, there is a strong rationale for recommending a physically active lifestyle for children, since it may help reduce risk factors for CVD and lower the CVD risk of a sedentary lifestyle as well as tracking to the increased likelihood of a physically active adulthood.

7.3   PHYSICAL ACTIVITY AND CARDIOVASCULAR FITNESS

There is a strong relationship between regular physical activity and cardiovascular fitness in youth and children both between the ages of 3–6 and 6–17. Increased physical activity can be achieved in a variety of ways, all of which have been shown to improve cardiovascular fitness (26–28). These include after-school interventions and organized training programs. The latter have been shown to improve cardiovascular fitness in children in more effective ways than general physical activity programs. These programs typically involve physical activity or exercise on three or more days a week for 30–60 minutes at 50–90% VO_2 max or heart rate (HR) max. The added benefit of childhood physical activity programs is that they set a positive habit that is likely to carry into adulthood.

7.4   PHYSICAL ACTIVITY AND MUSCULAR FITNESS

Regular physical activity programs have also been shown to improve muscular fitness (29). This is important for not only the activities of daily living but also the ability to pursue aerobic fitness activities with less risk of injury. It is for this reason that the PAGA 2018 Scientific Report expanded the recommendations from the 2008 Scientific Report (12). In the 2008 Physical Activity Guidelines, the recommendation was made for children and adolescents ages 6–17 to engage in 60 minutes or more of moderate to vigorous physical activity (MVPA) per day as well as three sessions of muscle strengthening exercises per week. These recommendations were further supported by increased studies that were conducted between 2008 and 2018. Just as in aerobic conditioning, muscular fitness achieved in childhood and adolescents is likely to carry over into the adult years (1).

7.5   BODY WEIGHT AND ADIPOSITY

The prevalence of childhood obesity has increased significantly since the 1980s paralleling the increased prevalence of obesity in adults over the same period of time. Regular physical activity can play an important role both to lower the risk of weight gain and to lower risk factors for chronic disease in children who are overweight or obese (30). The overall prevalence of childhood obesity appears to have plateaued near 18%. In the past decade comorbid conditions such as T2DM, dyslipidemia, and metabolic syndrome have also increased and are projected to continue to increase, unless ways can be found to slow the increase of childhood obesity. Children who are obese have also been shown to have reduced quality of life (31). Treating childhood obesity is challenging since many of the options available in adults are less available in children and many practicing clinicians report that they lack adequate training in treating childhood obesity.

Criteria for childhood obesity are as follows:

- Overweight (body mass index (BMI) ≥ 85th percentile through the 94th percentile for age and sex)
- Obese (BMI ≥ 95th percentile for age and sex)
- Severely obese (BMI > 120 percentile of 95th percentile or ≥ 35 kg/m^2).

An overall approach to treating childhood obesity is beyond the scope of this chapter; however, the role of physical activity is important and cannot be overstated. Multiple studies support that physical activity as an adjunct to nutritional and behavioral life-style interventions can result in small, short-term reductions in weight at very low risk. In addition, physical activity benefits in obese children and adolescents include improvements in vascular function, cardiorespiratory fitness, and cardiometabolic risk factors.

The PAGA 2018 Scientific Report recommends that 6–17-year-olds engage in at least 60 minutes per day in moderate to vigorous physical activities. These same guidelines apply to children who are overweight or obese. It should be emphasized that physical activity interventions in obese children are more likely to be successful if they are individualized to match baseline fitness/exercise tolerance level and also address stigma (e.g. weight-based teasing) that can have significant adverse effects on a child's body image, motivation, and desire to participate in any physical activity.

In addition, reduction in sedentary behavior is an essential and independent behavioral target for obesity treatment programs in children (17–19). (See subsequent section on sedentary behavior and health in children in this chapter and also Chapter 16 on sedentary behavior.) The PAGA 2018 Scientific Report rated high levels of physical activity as being associated with smaller increases in weight and adiposity during both childhood and adolescence (1).

7.6   BONE HEALTH

Multiple reviews of physical activity interventions including high impact, dynamic, short duration exercises such as hopping, skipping, jumping, and tumbling have been associated with increased bone mass and bone density (32–35). For this reason, the PAGA 2018 Scientific Report judged the evidence as strong for this type of regular physical activity for improving bone mass and density. Since children and adolescents are in the midst of their bone building years, this type of physical activity, particularly through weight bearing exercises, is extremely important to lower the subsequent risk of fractures and osteoporosis during adult years.

7.7   PHYSICAL ACTIVITY, SEDENTARY BEHAVIOR, AND HEALTH

Children and adolescents in the United States spend a substantial amount of time engaged in sedentary behaviors (17–21, 32–34). These behaviors include television viewing and other forms of "screen time" such as use of cell phones, tablets, and other devices for text messaging, playing video games, etc. In addition, there is time spent reading and studying at school and after school. It has been estimated that US children and adolescents spend 6–8 hours per day in sedentary behavior and that the majority spend more than 2 hours per day watching television or engaged in other types of screen time (32–34).

A number of studies have shown that sedentary behavior causes adverse health consequences. This includes some evidence that there is an association between sedentary behavior and increased cardiometabolic risk factors such as high blood pressure and dyslipidemia (36–38). There is also a strong association between TV or screen time and adiposity as well as a negative association between sedentary time and bone health outcomes (36–38). These data are of concern, since these relationships could result in ongoing health risks in adult life. For this reason, increasing physical activity represents an important mandate for youth. Since MVPA has been associated with multiple positive outcomes, replacing sedentary behavior with MVPA could significantly improve the health of American children and adolescents.

7.8 PHYSICAL ACTIVITY, COGNITIVE FUNCTION, AND ACADEMIC ACHIEVEMENT

Numerous studies have shown that increased physical activity positively affects cognitive function (39–40). Single bouts of physical activity intervention have been shown to improve short-term children's cognitive functioning. In addition, there are some data to suggest that increased physical activity is associated with improved academic achievement and engagement in school (41). Other research studies have shown that increased physical activity results in improvement in physical self-perception and enhanced self-esteem (42).

Recent advances in technology have allowed research to begin the exploration of how physical activity impacts on brain structure and function in youth. These studies typically involve magnetic resonance imaging. Early data have suggested that increased physical activity may modify white matter and activation of regions key to cognitive processes including executive function. Further research will be needed to clarify many of these preliminary findings.

7.9 PHYSICAL ACTIVITY AND FAMILY, SCHOOL, COMMUNITY, AND GOVERNMENT STRATEGIES

There is limited research available about the relationship between physical activity and the role that family and peers can play in this area. The 2016 United States of America Report Card on Physical Activity in Children and Youth rated information in this area as inconclusive (11).

Schools can represent an environment to potentially influence physical activity in many children and youth. Based on the data of the prevalence of high school students who attend at least one physical activity education class a week, only 48% of high school students achieve this. Participation in physical activity is higher in boys (53.3%) compared to girls (43.8%) and decreases across the high school years. Data from the School Health Policies and Practices Study in 2014 (43) show that the schools requiring physical education ranges from 43% to 47% from kindergarten to

5th grade and continues to decrease in the greatest fashion through 11th and 12th grade, where the percentage is below 9.

Community resources can also provide an opportunity for increased physical activity. The 2014 Report Card on Physical Activity in Youth demonstrated that 84.6% of children 12 years or younger live in neighborhoods with at least one park or playground area (43). Though this is a useful piece of information, it is only one of a number of aspects of the built environment that can influence the likelihood that children will improve or increase their physical activity.

Local state and federal governments also can play an important role in the promotion of physical activity among the children and youth. In the 2016 Report Card (11), data as how these government agencies are working in the area of physical activity was considered to be inconclusive. More information about the role of community and built environment for promoting physical activity may be found in Chapter 17.

7.10   CONCLUSIONS

Enormous data demonstrate that there are strong relationships between levels of physical activity and various health and fitness parameters in children. The most recent data in this area suggest that this is true not only for children and adolescents between the ages 6 and 17, which was reported in the 2008 PAGA, but now extends also to children 3–6 years of age.

The guidelines from the PAGA 2018 Scientific Report and the ACSM both recommend that children and youth obtain 60 minutes of MVPA on most, if not all, days and three sessions of musculoskeletal fitness each week. Unfortunately, 80% of children do not achieve these levels. Given the multiple benefits of regular physical activity for children and youth, this presents a big problem and suggests that future generations in the United States will suffer many needless health risks caused by insufficient levels of physical activity unless this is remedied. Moreover, increased technology has contributed to large amounts of sedentary behavior. This behavior, in turn, has led to increases in risk factors for cardiometabolic disease making it all the more incumbent upon clinicians to focus more attention on physical activity in youth.

CLINICAL APPLICATIONS

- Children in the United States and other developed countries are not achieving adequate levels of physical activity.
- Increased physical activity has been associated with multiple benefits including decreased risk factors for CVD and improved cardiovascular fitness and muscular fitness as well as decreased likelihood of obesity, improved bone health, and improved cognitive health.
- Conversely, sedentary behavior can increase the risk factors for adverse health consequences.
- All clinicians should assess levels of physical activity in children and youth and make recommendations based on the Physical Guidelines for Americans 2018 and the Position Statement of the ACSM. Recommended

levels of physical activity include 60 minutes of moderate or vigorous physical activity per day and three sessions of muscular fitness per week.

- Nearly 80% of children and adolescents do not achieve these recommended levels.
- All clinicians should assess and recommend levels of physical activity in children and adolescents.

REFERENCES

1. Physical Activity Guidelines Advisory Committee. 2018 Physical Activity Guidelines Advisory Committee. 2018 Scientific Report. Youth. Washington, DC: U.S. Department of Health and Human Services.
2. Andersen L, Murray R. Cardiovascular risk and physical activity in children. In Rippe JM (ed): Lifestyle Medicine (3rd edition). CRC Press (Boca Raton), 2019.
3. Ekelund U, Luan J, Sherar L, et al. Moderate to vigorous physical activity and sedentary time and cardiometabolic risk factors in children and adolescents. JAMA. 2012;307:704–712.
4. American College of Sports Medicine. http://www.acsm.org/docs/default-source/files-for-resource-library/physical-activity-in-children-and-adolescents.pdf?sfvrsn=be7978a7_2 [Accessed January 13, 2020].
5. Donnelly J, Hillman C, Castelli D, et al. Physical activity, fitness, cognitive function, and academic achievement in children: a systematic review. Med Sci Sports Exercise. 2016;48:1197–1222.
6. Centers for Disease Control and Prevention. Physical Activity for Everyone. http://www.cdc.gov/physicalactivity/everyone/guidelines/children.html [Accessed January 13, 2020].
7. Australian Government Department of Health and Ageing. Physical activity recommendations for 5-17 year olds. https://www1.health.gov.au/internet/main/publishing.nsf/Content/health-pubhlth-strateg-phys-act-guidelines#npa517 [Accessed January 13, 2020].
8. Canadian Society for Exercise Physiology. Canadian physical activity guidelines information sheet. http://www.csep.ca/english/view.asp?x=804 [Accessed January 13, 2020].
9. Department of Health. UK physical activity guidelines. https://www.gov.uk/government/collections/physical-activity-guidelines [Accessed January 13, 2020].
10. American Heart Association. The AHA's Recommendations for Physical Activity in children. http://www.heart.org/HEARTORG/HealthyLiving/PhysicalActivity/Physical-Activity-and-Children_UCM_304053_Article.jsp#.XjGvRk9Kios [Accessed January 29, 2020].
11. National Physical Activity Plan Alliance. The 2016 United States Report Card on Physical Activity for Children and Youth. Washington, DC: National Physical Activity Plan Alliance, 2016. https://www.physicalactivityplan.org/reportcard/2016FINAL_USReportCard.pdf [Accessed January 15, 2020].
12. US Department of Health and Human Services (USDHHS). Physical Activity Guidelines Advisory Committee Report, 2008. Washington, DC: USDHHS; 2008. US Department of Health and Human Services (USDHHS) https://health.gov/paguidelines/2008/pdf/paguide.pdf [Accessed January 15, 2020].
13. Erlandson M, Kontulainen S, Chilibeck PD, et al. Bone mineral accrual in 4- to 10-year-old precompetitive, recreational gymnasts: a 4-year longitudinal study. J Bone Miner Res. 2011;26(6):1313–1320. doi:10.1002/jbmr.338.
14. Janz K, Gilmore J, Burns T, et al. Physical activity augments bone mineral accrual in young children: the Iowa bone development study. J Pediatr. 2006;148(6):793–799.

15. Janz K, Letuchy E, Burns T, et al. Objectively measured physical activity trajectories predict adolescent bone strength: Iowa bone development study. Br J Sports Med. 2014;48(13):1032–1036. doi:10.1136/bjsports-2014-093574.

16. Gunter K, Almstedt H, Janz K. Physical activity in childhood may be the key to optimizing lifespan skeletal health. Exerc Sport Sci Rev. 2012;40(1):13–21. doi:10.1097/JES.0b013e318236e5ee.

17. Chinapaw M, Proper K, Brug J, et al. Relationship between young peoples' sedentary behaviour and biomedical health indicators: a systematic review of prospective studies. Obes Rev. 2011;12(7):e621–e632. doi:10.1111/j.1467-789X.2011.00865.x.

18. Tremblay M, LeBlanc A, Kho M, et al. Systematic review of sedentary behaviour and health indicators in school-aged children and youth. Int J Behav Nutr Phys Act. 2011;8:98. doi:10.1186/1479-5868-8-98.

19. Carson V, Hunter S, Kuzik N, et al. Systematic review of sedentary behaviour and health indicators in school-aged children and youth: an update. Appl Physiol Nutr Metab. 2016;41(6 suppl 3):S240–S265. doi:10.1139/apnm-2015-0630.

20. Cliff D, Hesketh K, Vella S, et al. Objectively measured sedentary behaviour and health and development in children and adolescents: systematic review and meta-analysis. Obes Rev. 2016;17(4):330–344. doi:10.1111/obr.12371.

21. Ried-Larsen M, Grontved A, Froberg K, et al. Physical activity intensity and subclinical atherosclerosis in Danish adolescents: the European youth heart study. Scand. J. Med. Sci. Sports. 2013;23(3): e168–e177.

22. Ried-Larsen M, Grontved A, Kristensen P, et al. Moderate-and-vigorous physical activity from adolescence to adulthood and subclinical atherosclerosis in adulthood: prospective observations from the European youth heart study. Br. J. Sports Med. 2015;49(2): 107–112.

23. Guinhouya B, Samouda H, Zitouni D, et al. Evidence of the influence of physical activity on the metabolic syndrome and/or on insulin resistance in pediatric populations: a systematic review. Int J Pediatr Obes. 2011;6(5-6):361–388.

24. Janssen I, Leblanc A. Systematic review of the health benefits of physical activity and fitness in school-aged children and youth. Int J Behav Nutr Phys Act. 2010;7:40. doi:10.1186/1479-5868-7-40.

25. Escalante Y, Saavedra J, García-Hermoso A, et al. Improvement of the lipid profile with exercise in obese children: a systematic review. Prev Med. 2012;54(5):293–301. doi:10.1016/j.ypmed.2012.02.006.

26. Beets MW, Beighle A, Erwin HE, Huberty JL. After-school program impact on physical activity and fitness: a meta-analysis. Am J Prev Med. 2009;36(6):527–537. doi:10.1016/j.amepre.2009.01.033.

27. Larouche R, Saunders T, Faulkner G, et al. Associations between active school transport and physical activity, body composition, and cardiovascular fitness: a systematic review of 68 studies. J Phys Act Health. 2014;11(1):206–227.

28. Sun C, Pezic A, Tikellis G, et al. Effects of school-based interventions for direct delivery of physical activity on fitness and cardiometabolic markers in children and adolescents: a systematic review of randomized controlled trials. Obes Rev. 2013;14(10):810–838.

29. Vasconcellos F, Seabra A, Katzmarzyk P, et al. Physical activity in overweight and obese adolescents: systematic review of the effects on physical fitness components and cardiovascular risk factors. Sports Med. 2014;(8):1139–1152.

30. Kelley GA, Kelley KS, Pate RR. Effects of exercise on BMI z-score in overweight and obese children and adolescents: a systematic review with meta-analysis. BMC Pediatr. 2014;14:225. doi:10.1186/1471-2431-14-225.

31. Moore J, Haemer M. Childhood obesity. In Rippe JM (ed): Lifestyle Medicine (3rd edition). CRC Press (Boca Raton), 2019.

32. Hind K, Burrows M. Weight-bearing exercise and bone mineral accrual in children and adolescents: a review of controlled trials. Bone. 2007;40:14–27. doi:10.1016/j.bone. 2006.07.006.

33. Julián-Almárcegui C, Gómez-Cabello A, Huybrechts I, et al. Combined effects of interaction between physical activity and nutrition on bone health in children and adolescents: a systematic review. Nutr Rev. 2015;73(3):127–139. doi:10.1093/nutrit/nuu065.

34. Tan V, Macdonald H, Kim S, et al. Influence of physical activity on bone strength in children and adolescents: a systematic review and narrative synthesis. J Bone Miner Res. 2014;29(10):2161–2181. doi:10.1002/jbmr.2254.

35. Weaver C, Gordon C, Janz K, et al. The national osteoporosis Foundation's position statement on peak bone mass development and lifestyle factors: a systematic review and implementation recommendations. Osteoporos Int. 2016 Apr;27(4):1281–1386.

36. LeBlanc A, Spence J, Carson V, et al. Systematic review of sedentary behaviour and health indicators in the early years (aged 0-4 years). Appl Physiol Nutr Metab. 2012;37(4):753–772. doi:10.1139/h2012-063.

37. Azevedo L, Ling J, Soos I, et al. The effectiveness of sedentary behaviour interventions for reducing body mass index in children and adolescents: systematic review and meta-analysis. Obes Rev. 2016;17(7):623–635. doi:10.1111/obr.12414.

38. Wu L, Sun S, He Y, et al. The effect of interventions targeting screen time reduction: a systematic review and meta-analysis. Medicine (Baltimore). 2016;95(27):e4029. doi:10.1097/MD.0000000000004029.

39. de Greeff J, Bosker R, Oosterlaan J, et al. Effects of physical activity on executive functions, attention and academic performance in preadolescent children: a meta-analysis. J Sci Med Sport. 2018;21:501–507.

40. Donnelly J, Hillman C, Castelli D, et al. Physical activity, fitness, cognitive function, and academic achievement in children: a systematic review. Med Sci Sports Exercise. 2016;48:1197–1222.

41. Owen K, Parker P, Van Zanden B, et al. Physical activity and school engagement in youth: a systematic review and meta-analysis. Educ Psychol. 2016;51:129–145.

42. Lubans D, Richards J, Hillman C, et al. Physical activity for cognitive and mental health in youth: a systematic review of mechanisms. Pediatrics. 2016;138:e20161642.

43. American Academy of Pediatrics Council on Communications and Media. Policy statement – children, adolescents, obesity and the media. Pediatrics. 2011;128:201–208.

8 Physical Activity in Older Adults

KEY POINTS

- Individuals over the age of 65 comprise approximately 13% of the adult population in the United States and are expected to grow to 19% of the total population by 2030. This is the most rapidly growing segment of the population.
- Physical activity conveys multiple benefits for individuals over the age of 65 including decreased risk of chronic disease or as an adjunct to its treatment, increased physical function, and decrease risk of falls.
- Increased physical activity may be particularly valuable for individuals who suffer from frailty or who have low levels of current physical activity.
- Unfortunately, only 27% of individuals over the age of 65 meet current recommendations for levels of physical activity.
- Clinicians should become knowledgeable about safe and effective ways of helping individuals over the age of 65 to increase levels of physical activity in their lives.

8.1   INTRODUCTION

In 2016 individuals over the age of 65 comprised approximately 13% of the United States population (1). Their numbers are projected to reach 72.1 million (19% of the total population) by year 2030 (2). This age group is the most rapidly growing of all population segments in the United States.

A large and persuasive body of scientific evidence supports the concept that regular physical activity yields multiple health and quality of life benefits for individuals over the age of 65 (3). Yet, despite the known health benefits of physical activity in this population, participation rates remain low with only 27% of adults over the age of 65 meeting recommended levels (4). Because of the aging of the population in the United States and elsewhere, finding cost-effective mechanisms for improving the health and forestalling disability in this age group, assumes great importance. The role of physical activity is central to the lifestyle measures for people over the age of 65 that can contribute to health, longevity, and improved quality of life.

Over the past decade, views of the population over the age of 65 have changed dramatically. This has also given rise to the concept of "successful aging" which has been promulgated by a number of investigators (5).

The purpose of the current chapter is to provide a summary of recent scientific information related to the role of physical activity in the elderly population. This body of scientific information has clearly demonstrated that physical activity improves physical function in individuals over the age of 65 as well as reducing the risks of chronic diseases or assist in their treatment if already present as well as lowering the risk of injuries related to falls and reducing the risk of developing chronic disability in the elderly population (1, 5, 6).

8.2 PHYSICAL ACTIVITY AND PHYSICAL FUNCTION IN OLDER ADULTS

The Physical Activity Guidelines for American Advisory Committee Scientific Report 2018 concluded that strong evidence supports that physical activity improves physical function and reduces age related loss of physical function in the aging population. The PAGA 2018 further reported that there was an inverse dose/response relationship between the volume of aerobic physical activity and the risk of physical function limitations in the aging population (1). According to the National Health Interviews Survey conducted between 2001 and 2007, 22.9% of older adults between the ages of 60 and 69 reported limitations such as great difficulty or inability to do the basic tasks of life (e.g., walk a quarter of a mile or lift a 10 pound bag of groceries etc.) (7). At the same time, 42.9% of adults aged 80 or older reported significant limitations in these areas. The 2008 Physical Activity Guidelines report concluded that physical activity could prevent or delay disability in individuals over the age of 65 (8). The evidence was rated as "moderate to strong." In the ensuing ten years before the PAGA 2018 Scientific Report was issued, the evidence had become increasingly persuasive of the important role of physical activity in limiting disability in this population.

Based on multiple studies conducted between 2008 and 2016, including randomized controlled trials (RCTs) and cohort studies of aerobic activity, muscle strengthening, balance and/or multicomponent physical activity programs, strong evidence was generated that physical activity improves physical function and reduces age-related loss of physical function in the general aging population (1). This evidence includes a variety of performance tests such as walking speed, balance measures, and self-reports of physical function and quality of life such as derived from the 36 item Short-Form survey (SF-36) physical functioning scale as well as the activity of daily living scales (3).

The PAGA 2018 also reported that meta-analyses and cohort studies provided strong evidence of a dose/response relationship between level and amount of physical activity and physical function as well as aerobic, muscle strengthening, and multicomponent physical activity (9). Some evidence was found that Tai Chi (10), yoga (11), Qijong (12), flexibility exercises and activities such as dancing and active video gaming may also improve physical functioning in the elderly population although the evidence in support of these latter activities is limited.

Cohort studies of physical activity in the aging population have suggested that approximately a 50% reduction in major functional limitations may occur in individuals who are regularly physically active. For example, individuals who are regularly physically active appear to be able to walk somewhat faster than individuals who are inactive (13). While minor changes in walking speed may seem like a small improvement, 10 year survival at the age of 75 varies across observed range of gait speeds from 19–87% in men and from 35–91% in women with significant improvements at as little as 0.1 meters per second of increased speed (14).

Physical function in older adults is extremely important from a public health standpoint given the rapidly increasing number of people over the age of 65. It should also be noted that the number of people over the age of 85 years old is projected to rise to 14.6 million by 2040 (2). Individuals in this age group also stand to derive significant functional improvements from regular physical activity as do the "frail" elderly.

8.3 PHYSICAL ACTIVITY AND FALL PREVENTION

Falls can present multiple medical challenges for individuals over the age of 65 and often herald the end of independent living. Regular physical activity has been demonstrated to decrease the likelihood of a fall. In fact, the PAGA 2018 concluded that there was strong evidence that multi-component physical activity exercise programs can significantly reduce the risk of injuries from falls including severe falls that may result in bone fracture, head trauma, open wound soft-tissue injury, or other injuries requiring medical care or admission to the hospital.

The PAGA 2018 cited results from systematic reviews and meta-analyses of RCTs which consistently supported that physical activity fall prevention programs reduce the risk of fall related injuries by 32–40% and bone fractures from 40–66% amongst individuals over the age of 65 (6,15–17). These RCT findings were also supported by three prospective cohort studies and one case control study.

The meta-analyses of RCTs also suggested that there is an inverse-response dose response relationship between the amount of moderate to vigorous physical activity and the magnitude of reduction of risk in fall related injuries and bone fractures. Three cohort and one case control study suggested that adults 65 years and older who participated in physical activity of at least moderate intensity for 30 minutes or more per day reduced the risk of fall related injuries and bone fracture (17). There is also evidence that even adults ages 85 and older obtain similar benefits from as little as 60 minutes or more per week at either a home or group-based physical activity programs.

The PAGA 2018 report cautioned that lower amounts of physical activity such as slow walking may not be sufficient to reduce the risk of fall related injury and bone fracture in the older population. The relationship between regular physical activity and the risk of fracture in older men is depicted in Figure 8.1.

This figure demonstrates a significant dose response relationship. Similar data are available related to the reduced risk of fall related injuries in women as well.

These results have significant public health implications. Up to 25% of individuals over the age of 65 years or older fall in the United States every year (1). In addition, falls are the leading cause of fatal injury and the most common cause of non-fatal trauma related hospital admissions for older adults. The effectiveness of physical activity programs to lower the risk of falls has significant public health relevance in the older age population because of the high prevalence of falls and related

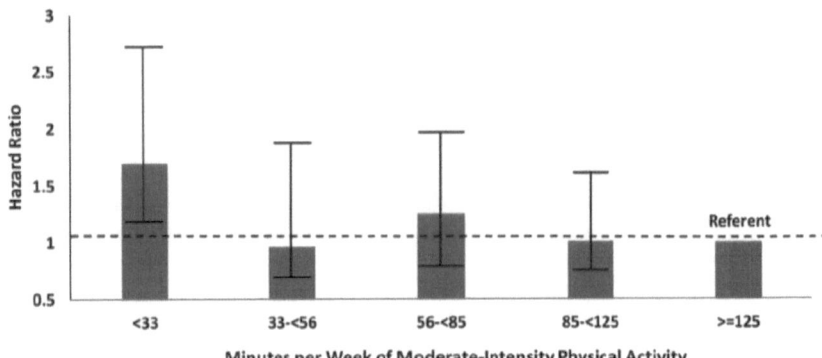

Minutes per Week of Moderate-Intensity Physical Activity

FIGURE 8.1   One-year risk of fracture in older men by quintile of moderate-intensity physical activity: the osteoporotic fractures in men study (N = 2,731).

Physical Activity Guidelines Advisory Committee. 2018 Physical Activity Guidelines Advisory Committee. 2018 Physical Activity Guidelines Advisory Committee Scientific Report. Older Adults. Washington, DC: U.S. Department of Health and Human Services (1). (From Cauley JA, Harrison SL, Cawthon PM, Ensrud KE, Danielson ME, Orwoll E, Mackey DC. Objective measures of physical activity, fractures and falls: the osteoporotic fractures in men study. J Am Geriatr Soc. 2013;61:1080–1088. doi:10.1111/jgs.12326.)

fall injuries and fractures in older adults often yielding increases in morbidity and disability and reduced quality of life.

8.4   PHYSICAL ACTIVITY AND COGNITIVE FUNCTION

Physical activity has been repeatedly demonstrated to improve cognitive function in individuals over the age of 65 (18). There is a known progressive, age-related decline in variety of aspects of the brain structure and function. For example, both cross sectional and longitudinal epidemiologic studies have estimated that the rate of decline in brain volume is about 0.3% per year resulting in average decrease of about 15% between the ages of 30 and 80 years of age (19). This may be associated also with decline of cognitive processes including memory, learning ability, problem solving and executive control.

Decreases in cognitive function in the aging brain may range from relatively minor changes to age related memory impairment (ARMI), mild cognitive impairment (MCI), and various forms of dementia including Alzheimer's Disease (20). Physical activity, especially aerobic exercise, of sufficient intensity and volume needed to increase aerobic fitness has been repeatedly demonstrated to result in improved cognitive function in people over the age of 65. The benefits are documented at 150–180 minutes per week of moderate intensity aerobic physical activity. Of course, these levels of increased physical activity also result in decrease risk of cardiovascular disease (CVD), type 2 diabetes (T2DM), and a variety of cancers (21–26).

A number of studies have shown that increased levels of physical activity at the levels recommended by ACSM and the PAGA 2018 also reduce the risk of both MCI and dementia (20). It has been speculated, based on animal work, that regular exercise is associated with increased brain derived neurotrophic factor (BDNF) (25), which promotes neurogenesis including the generation of new neurons and synapses. Both human and animal studies have also shown that exercise increases serum and cerebral spinal levels of insulin-like growth factor (IGF-1) (25), which also plays a significant role in brain function and cognition. Of course, aerobic exercise has well documented beneficial cardiovascular benefits which may include increased blood flow to the brain and decreased atherosclerosis in cerebral vessels. These issues are explored in greater detail in Chapter 11.

8.5 PHYSICAL ACTIVITY AND REDUCING AGE ASSOCIATED SARCOPENIA

Skeletal muscle mass and strength typically peak in the mid-20s to 30 years of age. There is generally a progressive decline of about 1% of every year up until the age of 70 after which the rate of muscle loss accelerates to about 2–3% per year (27, 28). Thus, during the aging process, a loss of over 30% of one's peak muscle mass may occur. This can eventually create significant problems in elderly individuals with the development of frailty.

The term "sarcopenia" refers to loss of skeletal muscle and functions attributed primarily to aging although it can also occur with extreme weight loss, cancer or other wasting disease conditions (29). Physical activity has been routinely shown to slow the process of progressive sarcopenia. Regular physical activity to slow the process of sarcopenia is important throughout the lifespan but appears to be most prominent after the age of 40–50 years. Recommendations for reducing the rate of muscle loss include the following (30):

- Resistance training 2–3 days per week of 8–10 upper and lower body exercises utilizing strength training machines, weight lifting, bands, or body weight.
- Moderate or vigorous aerobic/cardiorespiratory endurance training 3–5 days per week for 30–60 minutes per session including walking, stationary outdoor cycling, swimming, or other lower impact forms of aerobic physical activity.
- Flexibility or balance training to reduce the risk of falls and associated musculoskeletal injuries

Accumulating 150 minutes per week may further slow the process of age-related muscle loss. Theoretical reasons for slowing the process of age-related muscle loss through physical activity include the anti-inflammatory effects of regular activity, reduced oxidative stress, and enhanced quality and quantity of muscle protein, and mitochondrial function.

8.6 PHYSICAL ACTIVITY AND PHYSICAL FUNCTION IN OLDER ADULTS WITH SELECTED CHRONIC CONDITIONS

Increased physical activity can play a significant role in many of the chronic conditions which frequently occur in the elderly population. Specifically, the PAGA 2018 Scientific Report listed six of the most common conditions experienced in the elderly population and the role that physical activity plays reducing the risk or ameliorating each (1). More information about the role of physical activity in multiple chronic conditions may be found in Chapter 9.

- Cardiovascular disease—In individuals over the age of 65 with existing CVD, multiple studies have shown that either increased aerobic activity or strength training can yield significant functional benefits (31–33). In addition, as discussed in Chapters 3 and 9 increased physical activity can lower the risk of CVD across the lifespan.

    Chronic Obstructive Pulmonary Disease (COPD)—There is some evidence, although limited, that various forms of physical activity in individuals over the age of 50 result in functional improvement in such areas as walking ability (as measured by the six minute walk test) in older adults with COPD (34–35).

- Cognitive impairment—The issue of cognitive function is of great importance to the elderly population (36–39). Approximately 20–30% of adults over the age of 65 suffer from either mild cognitive impairment or dementia. Decreases in physical function can often exist in addition to cognitive losses and accelerate the risk of the need for care giving. The scientific literature has demonstrated that both measures of physical function and cognition can increase with physical activity in individuals over the age of 65. More detail concerning the role of physical activity in cognition across the lifespan may be found in Chapter 11.

- Frailty—Multiple systematic reviews and meta-analyses have reported that physical activity lowers the risk of frailty and improves some or all measures of physical function in older people who already have frailty. (See Chapter 9.)

- Hip fracture—Hip fracture is a significant health risk in individuals over the age of 65 (40). Measurements of physical activity programs following hip fracture have typically demonstrated beneficial effects in function for older adults. The most common form of physical activity involves muscle strengthening exercises although in some instances the physical activity trials also involved other modes of activity. (See Chapter 9.)

    Osteoporosis or osteopenia—Significant improvements in self-reported physical function in individuals with osteoporosis or osteopenia over the age of 65 have been demonstrated in individuals who are involved in programs of increased physical activity in areas such as strengthening, stretching, agility, and/or balance training (41–43). In this area, programs that combine strength training with agility and balance training appear to improve physical function scores more than programs which involve only strength training. (See also Chapter 9.)

- Parkinson's disease—A variety of programs with different modes of physical activity have been employed in individuals with Parkinson's disease (44–46). These programs have typically shown small to moderate improvements in a variety of physical function measurements including gait velocity, the 6 minute walk and "timed up and go" and balance score and strength. (See also Chapter 9.)

- Stroke—Evidence of benefits of physical activity following stroke is based on individuals who have survived a stroke and are still able to walk at a walking speed of at least 0.3 meters per second (47, 48). Physical activity modalities in these individuals involve primarily strength and mobility training. Improvements in walking function in older people following a stroke with the evidence of this area reported in the PAGA 2018 rated as "moderate." (See Chapter 9.)
- Visual impairments—Older individuals with visual impairments may have particularly greater age-related problems with balance than individuals without visual impairments (49). There are few reported studies that evaluate physical activity in these adults.

8.7   OVERALL PUBLIC HEALTH IMPACT

Chronic conditions are very prevalent in adults over the age of 65. It has been estimated that approximately 80% of adults over the age of 70 have one chronic condition and 77% have at least two chronic diseases resulting in 75% of heath care spending in the United States (50). There is strong evidence that indicates that physical inactivity is a strong predictor of physical disability in older people. Given that the percentage of individuals over the age of 65 is rapidly growing in the United States physical activity may be a particularly promising option for older individuals with established chronic conditions.

8.8   PHYSICAL ACTIVITY AND SUCCESSFUL AGING

Given the rapidly increasing number of individuals over the age of 65, finding ways to help older individuals decrease health problems associated with aging and lead high quality lives has assumed significant importance (5). This is particularly important because of a number of studies including the Health and Retirement Study found that only 11.9% of older individuals were categorized as "aging successfully" (51). This has led to interest in the concept of "successful aging."

One of the most prominent models of successful aging was developed by Rowe and Khan (52, 53). The framework of successful aging defined by these investigators included a low risk of disease and disease related disability, high mental and physical function, and active engagement with life (52, 53). In order to be categorized as "aging successfully" individuals in these studies had to display high levels in all three of these characteristics. The role of physical activity is very important in all three of these areas, particularly in individuals over the age of 65. Indeed, increased physical activity has the potential to serve as the primary vehicle of enhancing and maintaining each of these three characteristics (54–56).

As already indicated, increased physical activity is highly important to help older individuals maintain physical function, decrease the likelihood of falling, slow the process of cognitive decline (57–-59), and reduce age-associated muscle loss (sarcopenia) (18). These areas are important to elderly individuals who are healthy and also who have chronic conditions.

Importantly, the concept of successful aging has helped scientists understand the types of factors needed to improve quality of life in the elderly population. This can help reverse the common misconception that older age is simply a period of inevitable decline.

8.9   PRESCRIBING PHYSICAL ACTIVITY FOR OLDER ADULTS

Given the multiple demonstrated benefits of increased physical activity for older adults it is incumbent on physicians to become knowledgeable about how to prescribe increased physical activity for this age group.

The recommendations for physical activity levels in older adults are very similar to younger individuals (1). Specifically, it is recommended that to achieve maximum benefit, 150–300 minutes of moderate intensity physical activity each week be conducted in sessions of at least ten minutes in duration. In addition, strength training activities two times a week utilizing the major muscle groups are also recommended as is balance training for all older adults. Avoiding sedentary activity is also very important for older adults. It is important to note that with only 27% of individuals over the age of 65 meet these criteria (1).

Individuals who have not been this active or who are truly sedentary should start at significantly lower levels than healthy younger individuals and progress slowly using symptoms as their guide.

A key issue for clinicians to consider is how to motivate older adults to maintain a physically active lifestyle and find ways of providing social support from family and friends which has been associated with long-term exercise adherence in older adults. It is important to emphasize how to incorporate active choices into daily life for individuals of all age groups but particularly in the older population. Discussions about how to perform physical activity in the safest way possible are also important for physicians to emphasize in individuals in the older population particularly if they have been sedentary (60).

8.10   PUBLIC HEALTH IMPLICATIONS

Increased physical activity has been demonstrated in multiple studies to offer significant benefits to the older population. These include significant improvements in physical function and a 30–40% reduction in the risk of falls (15–17). In addition, increased physical activity plays an important role in preserving cognitive function and decreasing the risk of cognitive impairment (18). Physical activity also is a central component in the emerging concept of "successful aging" (52, 53). Increased physical activity may be particularly important in individuals who have limitations in physical function or chronic conditions. Not only aerobic conditioning but also strength training and balance training can all play important roles in the maintenance of an active healthy lifestyle in individuals over the age of 65. Physical activity may be particularly important for improving physical function in older adults who suffer from frailty. Increased physical activity has been shown in a number of studies to reduce the age related loss of muscle and thus can carry multiple health and functional benefits (29).

8.11 CONCLUSIONS

Given the multiple benefits of physical activity for individuals over the age of 65, it is important that every clinician emphasize increasing physical activity in the elderly population. This is particularly true since only 27% of individuals over the age of 65 meet the criteria of at least 150 of moderate intensity physical activity and two sessions of strength training per week. Given the rapidly increasing population of individuals over the age of 65, it is imperative that cost-effective ways of lowering health risks and improving physical function are developed in this age population. Physical activity offers one of the most powerful and cost effective ways of improving the health and quality of life in individuals over the age of 65.

CLINICAL APPLICATIONS

- Physical activity plays an important role in multiple aspects of health and well-being in individuals over the age of 65.
- Increased physical activity has been shown to be important to improve physical function, reduce the risk of falls, improve cognitive function, and reduce age-related decline in muscle mass.
- Recommended levels of physical activity for individuals over the age of 65 include at least 150 minutes per week of moderate intensity aerobic activity and 2–3 sessions of strength training per week as well as balance exercises.
- Clinicians should assess the current level of physical activity in their patients over the age of 65 and recommend ways of increasing safe and effective physical activity.
- Increased physical activity represents one of the most cost-effective and powerful ways of improving the health and well-being of individuals over the age of 65.
- The concept of "successful aging" can help clinicians understand the opportunities for individuals over the age of 65 to improve both their health and quality of life.

REFERENCES

1. Physical Activity Guidelines Advisory Committee. 2018 Physical Activity Guidelines Advisory Committee. 2018 Physical Activity Guidelines Advisory Committee Scientific Report. Older Adults. Washington, DC: U.S. Department of Health and Human Services.
2. Administration on Aging. U.S. Department of Health and Human Services. A profile of older Americans: 2016. Washington, DC: U.S. Department of Health and Human Services; 2016.
3. Pahor M, Guralnik J, Ambrosius W, et al. Effect of structured physical activity on prevention of major mobility disability in older adults: the LIFE study randomized clinical trial. JAMA. 2014;311(23):2387–2396. doi:10.1001/jama.2014.5616.
4. Keadle S, McKinnon R, Graubard B, et al. Prevalence and trends in physical activity among older adults in the United States: a comparison across three national surveys. Prev Med. Aug. 2016;89:37–43. doi:10.1016/j.ypmed.2016.05.009.

5. Rose D. Aging successfully: Predictors and pathways. In Rippe JM (ed): Lifestyle Medicine (3rd edition). CRC Press (Boca Raton), 2019.
6. El-Khoury F, Cassou B, Charles MA, et al. The effect of fall prevention exercise programmes on fall induced injuries in community dwelling older adults: systematic review and meta-analysis of randomised controlled trials. BMJ. 2013;347:f6234. doi: 10.1136/bmj.f6234.
7. Holmes J, Powell-Griner E, Lethbridge-Cejku M, et al. Aging differently: physical limitations among adults aged 50 years and over: United States, 2001-2007. NCHS Data Brief. July 2009;(20):1–8.
8. Physical Activity Guidelines Advisory Committee. Physical Activity Guidelines Advisory Committee Report, 2008. Washington, DC: U.S. Department of Health and Human Services; 2008. https://health.gov/paguidelines/guidelines/report.aspx. Published 2008 [Accessed January 16, 2020].
9. Chase J, Phillips L, Brown M. Physical activity intervention effects on physical function among community-dwelling older adults: a systematic review and meta-analysis. J Aging Phys Act. 2017;25(1):149–170. doi:10.1123/japa.2016-0040
10. Leung D, Chan C, Tsang H, et al. Tai chi as an intervention to improve balance and reduce falls in older adults: a systematic and meta-analytical review. Altern Ther Health Med. 2011;17(1):40–48.
11. Youkhana S, Dean C, Wolff M, et al. Yoga-based exercise improves balance and mobility in people aged 60 and over: a systematic review and meta-analysis. Age Ageing. 2016;45(1):21–29. doi:10.1093/ageing/afv175.
12. Rogers C, Larkey L, Keller C. A review of clinical trials of tai chi and qigong in older adults. West J Nurs Res. 2009;31(2):245–279. doi:10.1177/0193945908327529
13. Hortobágyi T, Lesinski M, Gäbler M, et al. Effects of three types of exercise interventions on healthy old adults' gait speed: a systematic review and meta-analysis. Sports Med. 2015;45(12):1627–1643. doi:10.1007/s40279-015-0371-2.
14. Studenski S, Perera S, Patel K, et al. Gait speed and survival in older adults. JAMA. 2011;305(1):50–58. doi:10.1001/jama.2010.1923.
15. Gillespie L, Robertson M, Gillespie W, et al. Interventions for preventing falls in older people living in the community. Cochrane Database Syst Rev. 2012;9:CD007146. doi:10.1002/14651858.CD007146.pub3.
16. Zhao R, Feng F, Wang X. Exercise interventions and prevention of fall-related fractures in older people: a meta-analysis of randomized controlled trials. Int J Epidemiol. 2016. doi: 10.1093/ije/dyw142.
17. Health Quality Ontario. Prevention of falls and fall-related injuries in community-dwelling seniors: an evidence-based analysis. Ont Health Technol Assess Ser. 2008;8:1–78.
18. Leon A. Aging-associated cognitive decline and its attenuation by lifestyle. In Rippe JM (ed): Lifestyle Medicine (3rd edition). CRC Press (Boca Raton), 2019.
19. Raz N, Rodrigue K. Differential aging of the brain: patterns, cognitive correlates, and modifiers. Neurosci Biobehav Rev. 2006;30:730–748.
20. Fillit H, Butler R, O'Connell A, et al. Achieving and maintaining cognitive vitality with aging. Mayo Clinic Proc. 2002;77:681–696.
21. Fluza-Luces C, Garathachea N, Bergen N, et al. Exercise is the real polypill. Physiology. 2013;28:330–358.
22. Bherer L, Erickson K, Liu-Ambrose T. A review of the effects of physical activity and exercise on cognitive and brain functions in older adults. J Aging Res. 2013;2013:657508.
23. Lautenschlager N. The influence of exercise on brain aging and dementia. Biochem Biophys Acta. 2012;1822:474–481.
24. Lista I, Sorrentine G. Biological mechanisms of physical activity in preventing cognitive decline. Cell Mol Neurolbiol. 2010;30:493–503.
25. Barnes J. Exercise, cognitive function and aging. Adv Physiol Educ. 2015;39:55–62.

26. Colcombe S, Kramer A. Fitness effects as cognitive function of older adults: a meta-analysis study. Psychol Sci. 2003;14:125–130.
27. Leon A. Reducing aging-associated risk of sarcopenia. In Rippe JM (ed): Lifestyle Medicine (3rd edition). CRC Press (Boca Raton), 2019.
28. Leon A. Attenuation of adverse effects of aging on skeletal muscle by regular exercise and nutritional support. Am J Lifestyle Med. 2015;9:1–13.
29. Rosenberg I. Sarcopenia: origins and clinical relevance. J. Nutr. 1997;137:900S–9915.
30. Ji L., Gomez-Cabrera M, Vina, J. Exercise and hormesis activation of cellular antioxidant signaling pathway. Ann NY Acad Sci. 2006;1067:425–435.
31. Floegel T, Perez G. An integrative review of physical activity/exercise intervention effects on function and health-related quality of life in older adults with heart failure. Geriatr Nurs. 2016;37(5):340–347. doi:10.1016/j.gerinurse.2016.04.013.
32. Chen Y, Hunt M, Campbell K, et al. The effect of tai chi on four chronic conditions—cancer, osteoarthritis, heart failure and chronic obstructive pulmonary disease: a systematic review and meta-analyses. Br J Sports Med. 2016;50(7):397–407. doi:10.1136/bjsports-2014-094388.
33. Wang X, Pi Y, Chen P, et al. Traditional Chinese exercise for cardiovascular diseases: systematic review and meta-analysis of randomized controlled trials. J Am Heart Assoc. 2016;5(3):e002562. doi:10.1161/JAHA.115.002562.
34. Desveaux L, Beauchamp M, Goldstein R, et al. Community-based exercise programs as a strategy to optimize function in chronic disease: a systematic review. Med Care. 2014;52(3):216–226. doi:10.1097/MLR.000000000000006.
35. Iepsen U, Jørgensen K, Ringbaek T, et al. A systematic review of resistance training versus endurance training in COPD. J Cardiopulm Rehabil Prev. 2015;35(3):163–172. doi:10.1097/HCR.000000000000010.
36. Blankevoort C, van Heuvelen M, Boersma F, et al. Review of effects of physical activity on strength, balance, mobility and ADL performance in elderly subjects with dementia. Dement Geriatr Cogn Disord. 2010;30(5):392–402. doi:10.1159/000321357.
37. Brett L, Traynor V, Stapley P. Effects of physical exercise on health and well-being of individuals living with a dementia in nursing homes: a systematic review. J Am Med Dir Assoc. 2016;17(2):104–116. doi:10.1016/j.jamda.2015.08.016.
38. Pitkälä K, Savikko N, Poysti M, et al. Efficacy of physical exercise intervention on mobility and physical functioning in older people with dementia: a systematic review. Exp Gerontol. 2013;48(1):85–93. doi:10.1016/j.exger.2012.08.008.
39. Forbes D, Forbes S, Blake C, et al. Exercise programs for people with dementia. Cochrane Database Syst Rev. 2015;(4):Cd006489. doi:10.1002/14651858. CD006489.pub4.
40. Auais M, Eilayyan O, Mayo N. Extended exercise rehabilitation after hip fracture improves patients' physical function: a systematic review and meta-analysis. Phys Ther. 2012;92(11):1437–1451. doi:10.2522/ptj.20110274.
41. Giangregorio L, Macintyre N, Thabane L, et al. Exercise for improving outcomes after osteoporotic vertebral fracture. Cochrane Database Syst Rev. 2013;(1):Cd008618. doi:10.1002/14651858.CD008618.pub2.
42. Li W, Chen Y, Yang R, et al. Effects of exercise programmes on quality of life in osteoporotic and osteopenic postmenopausal women: a systematic review and meta-analysis. Clin Rehabil. 2009;23(10):888–896. doi:10.1177/0269215509339002.
43. Wilhelm M, Roskovensky G, Emery K, et al. Effect of resistance exercises on function in older adults with osteoporosis or osteopenia: a systematic review. Physiother Can. 2012;64(4):386–394. doi:10.3138/ptc.2011-31BH.
44. Alves Da Rocha P, McClelland J, Morris ME. Complementary physical therapies for movement disorders in Parkinson's disease: a systematic review. Eur J Phys Rehabil Med. 2015;51(6):693–704.

45. Brienesse L, Emerson M. Effects of resistance training for people with Parkinson's disease: a systematic review. J Am Med Dir Assoc. 2013;14(4):236–241. doi:10.1016/j.jamda.2012.11.012.

46. Crizzle A, Newhouse I. Is physical exercise beneficial for persons with Parkinson's disease? Clin J Sport Med. 2006;16(5):422–425.

47. Eng J, Tang P. Gait training strategies to optimize walking ability in people with stroke: a synthesis of the evidence. Expert Rev Neurother. 2007;7(10):1417–1436. doi:10.1586/14737175.7.10.1417.

48. Nascimento L, de Oliveira C, Ada L, et al. Walking training with cueing of cadence improves walking speed and stride length after stroke more than walking training alone: a systematic review. J Physiother. 2015;61(1):10–15. doi:10.1016/j.jphys.2014.11.015.

49. Gleeson M, Sherrington C, Keay L. Exercise and physical training improve physical function in older adults with visual impairments but their effect on falls is unclear: a systematic review. J Physiother. 2014;60(3):130–135. doi:10.1016/j.jphys.2014.06.010.

50. National Council on Aging. Fact sheet: healthy aging. https://www.ncoa.org/news/resources-forreporters/get-the-facts/healthy-aging-facts [Accessed January 16, 2020]. Arlington, VA: National Council on Aging; 2016.

51. McLaughlin S, Connell C, Heeringa S, et al. Successful aging in the United States: prevalence estimates from a national sample of older adults. J Gerontol Psychol Sci Soc Sci. 2009;65B(2):216–226.

52. Rowe J, Kahn R. Human aging: usual and successful. Science. 1987;237:143–149.

53. Rowe J, Kahn R. Successful Aging. Dell Publishing (New York), 1998.

54. Nelson M, Rejeski W, Blair S, et al. Physical activity and public health in older adults: recommendation from the American College of sports medicine and the American heart association. Med Sci Sports Exer. 2007;39:1435–1445.

55. Keysor J. Does late-life physical activity or exercise prevent or minimize disablement? A critical review of the scientific evidence. Am J Prev Med. 2003;25:129–136.

56. Baker J, Meisner B, Logan A, et al. Physical activity and successful aging in Canadian older adults. J Aging Phys Act. 2009;17:223–235.

57. Colcombe S, Kramer A. Fitness effects on the cognitive function of older adults: a meta-analytic study. Psychol Sci. 2003;14:125–130.

58. Hillman C, Belopolsky A, Snook E, et al. Physical activity and executive control: implications for increased cognitive health during older adulthood. Res Quart Exer Sport. 2004;75:176– 185.

59. Bixby W, Spalding T, Haufler A, et al. The unique relation of physical activity to executive function in older men and women. Med Sci Sports Exer. 2007;39:1408–1416.

60. Schwingel A, Chodzko-Zajko W. Role of physical activity in the health and wellbeing of older adults. In Rippe JM (ed): Lifestyle Medicine (3rd edition). CRC Press (Boca Raton), 2019.

9 Physical Activity in Individuals with Chronic Conditions

KEY POINTS

- Chronic conditions are prevalent in the American population.
- Over 50% of adults in the United States have at least one chronic condition.
- Increased physical activity has been shown to yield multiple benefits to individuals with a wide variety of chronic conditions.
- These benefits include improvements in physical function and health related quality of life as well as reduction of risk of co-morbid conditions.

9.1 INTRODUCTION

Chronic conditions are very common in the US population (1). Over half of Americans (51.7%) have at least one chronic condition and about one third (31.5%) have multiple chronic conditions (2). The prevalence of chronic conditions increases with age. About 80% of adults over the age of 65 or older have multiple chronic conditions (3). A listing of the most common chronic conditions in the United States in adults and children is found in Figure 9.1.

Physical Activity can play an important role for individuals who have chronic conditions. It can assist in the therapy of a chronic condition such as in formal rehabilitation programs. Physical activity can also lower the risk of developing chronic conditions and play an important role in reducing likelihood of comorbid conditions in individuals with chronic conditions (1, 4). Moreover, physical activity can play an important role in preventing chronic conditions from getting worse over time.

The purpose of the current chapter is to provide a summary of the most common chronic conditions in adults in the United States and outline the multiple important roles that increased physical activity can play in ameliorating or treating them. Some of these chronic conditions such as cancer, hypertension, diabetes, and multiple sclerosis are also discussed in more detail in other chapters in this book.

9.2 PHYSICAL ACTIVITY IN CANCER SURVIVORS

According to the U.S. National Cancer Institute, a person is considered to be a cancer survivor from the time of diagnosis until the end of life. Currently there are approximately 15 million people in the United States who are considered cancer survivors (5). Improvements in treatments and detection of cancer have contributed to increased survival. Most of the studies have been done in physical activity and in

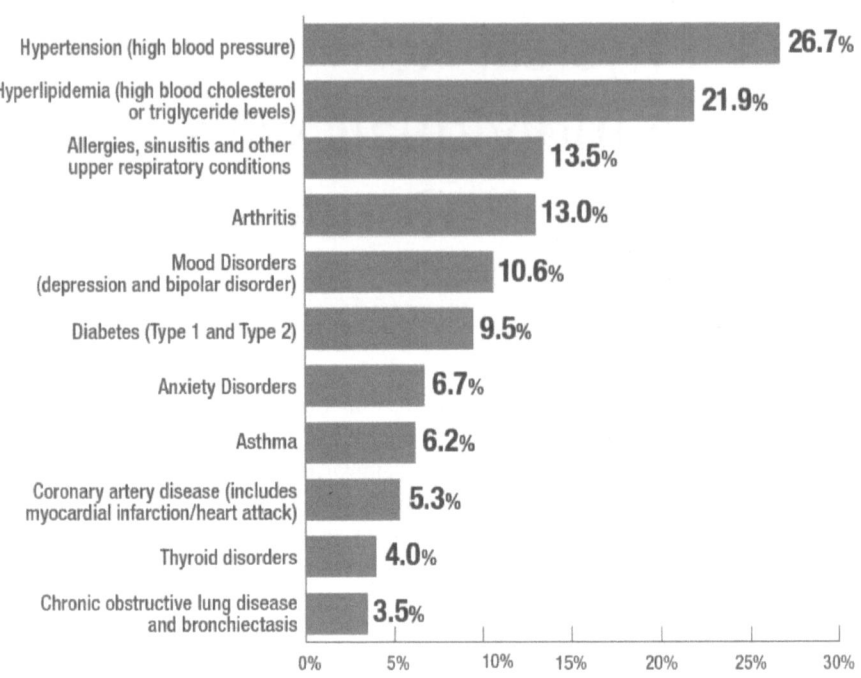

FIGURE 9.1   Most prevalent chronic conditions in adults and children, 2010.

(Physical Activity Guidelines Advisory Committee. 2018 Physical Activity Guidelines Advisory Committee. 2018 Physical Activity Guidelines Advisory Committee Scientific Report. Individuals with Chronic Conditions. Washington, DC: U.S. Department of Health and Human Services; 2018.) (From Gerteis J, Izrael D, Deitz D, et al. Multiple chronic conditions chartbook. AHRQ Publications No, Q14-0038. Rockville, MD: Agency for Healthcare Research and Quality; April 2014.)

cancer survival have been done on individual cancers since there is a great diversity of types of cancers and their underlying mechanisms.

Perhaps the most evidence regarding physical activity in cancer survivors is available in the area of breast cancer where greater amounts of physical activity after diagnosis are associated with lower risk of breast cancer specific mortality and all-cause mortality. This benefit has been demonstrated both in pre and postmenopausal breast cancer survivors. The role of physical activity in cancer survivors is particularly important since more than three million US women are living with the diagnosis of breast cancer (6).

In the area of colorectal cancer there is moderate evidence that increased levels of physical activity after diagnosis are associated with lower risk of colorectal cancer specific mortality and all-cause mortality. More than 1,300,000 individuals are colorectal cancer survivors (7, 8). Colorectal cancer accounts for about 52,600 deaths per year in the United States.

In prostate cancer survivors there is also some evidence of an inverse relationship between the highest and lowest levels of physical activity after diagnosis and all-cause mortality. More than 3,000,000 U.S. men are living with the diagnosis of invasive prostate cancer (9). As with many other cancers, prognosis is influenced by the stage at diagnosis and availability and access to appropriate therapies. The leading cause of death in older individuals with prostate cancer is cardiovascular disease (CVD).

The role of physical activity in overall cancer treatment and prognosis for many different cancers is important for a variety of reasons. It is estimated that 42% of men and 38% of women will develop cancer during their lifetimes (10). As therapies have continued to improve, the number of years that affected individuals will live continues to increase. Many cancer survivors can expect to live for decades after the diagnosis (11). With this body of information, the literature that supports an inverse relationship between greater levels of physical activity and decreased all-cause mortality and cancer specific mortality plays a very important role.

The Physical Activity Guidelines for Americans 2018 Scientific Advisory Report supported the recommendations for breast, colorectal, and prostate cancer survivors to increase physical activity (1). There are less data available in other cancers but this is an area of ongoing research. For all of these reasons, increased physical activity should be encouraged in survivors of breast, prostate, or colorectal cancer.

9.3 OSTEOARTHRITIS

Various arthritic conditions are prevalent in the US population. Arthritis affects over fifty four million Americans (12). Osteoarthritis (OA) is the most common joint disorder in the United States, affecting an estimated 30.8 million adults.

It is highly likely that the real burden of OA has been underestimated (13). OA of the knee and hip is the leading cause of mobility impairment in older adults in the United States. While OA is more common in older adults, it also can affect a wide spectrum of age groups. For example, two million Americans under the age of 45 have knee arthritis (14). As the population continues to age it is expected that the prevalence of OA will continue to grow. Some estimates have indicated there may be 74 million individuals with OA by the year 2040. This represents almost 26% of the total population of adults over the age of 18 (15).

Regular physical activity can yield significant benefits for people with OA. The current guidance from the PAGA 2018 Scientific Report recommends 150 minutes per week of moderate intensity aerobic exercise and two days a week of muscle strengthening exercise for individuals with OA. These levels of activities can generate substantial benefits for the overall population with pre-existing osteoarthritis. Benefits of physical activity in individuals with OA include decreased pain and improved physical function as well as improved health related quality of life, slower rates of disease progression and decreased likelihood of comorbid conditions (1,4).

9.4 PHYSICAL ACTIVITY AND HYPERTENSION

Hypertension is the most common and preventable risk factor for cardiovascular disease (CVD) (16). Data from the 2017 American College of Cardiology (ACC)/AHA Guidelines for the Prevention, Detection, and Evaluation and Management of High

Blood Pressure estimates that 46% of adults in the United States have high blood pressure utilizing the criteria of SBP/DBP ≥130 over ≥ 80 mm Hg (17).

According to the Framingham Heart Study, over 90% of adults who are free of hypertension at age 55 or 65 years will develop hypertension during their lifetime. It is estimated that for every 10 mm Hg increase in diastolic blood pressure or 20 mm Hg increase in systolic blood pressure above 120 over 75 mm Hg results in a doubling of the risk of heart disease (16). Hypertension is a significant risk factor for cardiovascular disease (CVD). High blood pressure is second only to cigarette smoking as a preventable cause of death for any reason (17). Regular physical activity conveys multiple health related benefits for individuals with hypertension.

There are multiple health related benefits for increased physical activity in individuals who have high blood pressure. These benefits include lowering blood pressure. As shown in Figure 9.2.

Regular aerobic physical activity can result in lowering of systolic blood pressure of approximately 8 mm Hg and lowering of diastolic blood pressure of approximately 6 mm Hg (18). Both of these represent significant reductions. Control of high blood pressure also lowers the risk of CVD and reduces the likelihood of progression of high blood pressure itself. In addition, regular physical activity can improve health related quality of life and increase physical function in individuals with high blood pressure (18). For all of these reasons, regular physical activity at the level of general recommendations from the PAGA 2018 Scientific Report is highly desirable in individuals with hypertension.

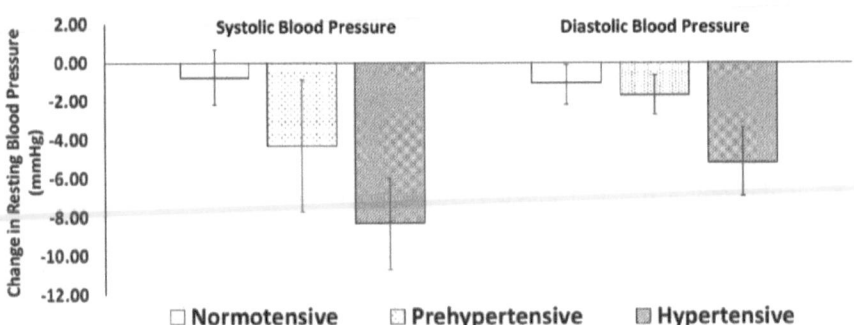

FIGURE 9.2 Blood pressure response to 16 weeks of aerobic physical activity, by resting blood pressure level.

Physical Activity Guidelines Advisory Committee. 2018 Physical Activity Guidelines Advisory Committee. 2018 Physical Activity Guidelines Advisory Committee Scientific Report. Washington, DC: U.S. Department of Health and Human Services; 2018 (1). (Adapted from Cornelissen VA, Smart NA. Exercise training for blood pressure: a systematic review and meta-analysis. J Am Heart Assoc. 2013;2(1):e004473. doi:10.1161/ JAHA.112.004473.)

9.5   PHYSICAL ACTIVITY AND TYPE 2 DIABETES (T2DM)

T2DM is prevalent in the population with over 9% of the population currently diagnosed with this condition (19). Physical Activity can play multiple positive health related roles in individuals with T2DM. For example, the leading cause of death in people with T2DM is CVD. Physical activity is associated with a 30–40% reduction in the risk of CVD mortality in individuals with T2DM (20).

There is a dose/response relationship with increasing levels of physical activity, lowering both the risk of CVD and CVD mortality in individuals with T2MD. In addition, regular physical activity can improve physical function and health related quality of life in individuals with T2DM (21).

Importantly, there is substantial evidence of an association between aerobic activity, muscle strengthening activity, and the combination of these two modalities with disease progression in people with T2DM including Hb-A1C, blood pressure, body mass index, and lipids.

There is a dose response relationship between physical activity and cardiovascular disease mortality in individuals with T2DM (22). This is illustrated in Figure 9.3.

As shown in Figure 9.3 there is an approximately 40% decrease in CVD mortality from individuals with T2DM who meet the PAGAC 2018 guidelines of 150 to 300 minutes of moderate to vigorous physical activity per week (23). Even

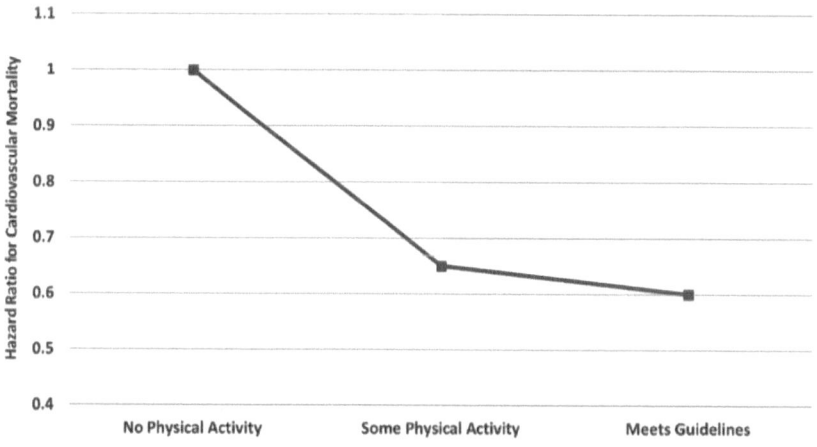

FIGURE 9.3   Dose-response relationship between physical activity and cardiovascular disease mortality in individuals with type 2 diabetes.

Physical Activity Guidelines Advisory Committee. 2018 Physical Activity Guidelines Advisory Committee. 2018 Physical Activity Guidelines Advisory Committee Scientific Report. Washington, DC: U.S. Department of Health and Human Services; 2018. (Adapted from Sadarangani K, Hamer M, Mindell J, et al. Physical activity and risk of all-cause and cardiovascular disease mortality in diabetic adults from Great Britain: Pooled analysis of 10 population-based cohorts. Diabetes Care. 2014;37:1016–1023.)

individuals who have some regular physical activity, but do not meet guidelines in individuals with T2DM, have their cardiovascular mortality reduced by 30%. For all of these reasons, there is strong evidence that increased levels of physical activity play multiple important health related roles in individuals with T2DM.

Finally, regular physical activity in addition to modest weight loss (5–7%), has been shown to lower the risk in individuals with prediabetes progressing to diabetes. In the Diabetes Prevention Program the combination of 150 minutes of daily moderate to vigorous physical activity plus 5–7% of weight loss resulted in to 58% decrease in the likelihood of T2DM (24). These reductions in risk are particularly significant given that 36–38% of individuals in the United States have prediabetes (25). More information related to the role of physical activity in diabetes and prediabetes may be found in Chapter 5.

9.6 MULTIPLE SCLEROSIS

Individuals with multiple sclerosis (MS) are typically less active than comparably aged populations without this condition. Regular physical activity can improve multiple aspects of health in individuals with MS (26, 27). For example, regular physical activity has the potential to improve physical function in these individuals. One frequent health benefit of increased physical activity involves improved mobility in such areas as slight increases in walking speed. The type of physical activity recommended typically involves both aerobic and muscle strengthening activities in addition to improving walking speed. Endurance is also improved by increased physical activity.

Other benefits of regular physical activity in individuals with MS include improvements in health related quality of life. Regular physical activity may also lower the risk of comorbid conditions, although few research trials have been conducted in this area. With regard to health related quality of life, in addition to overall improvements in this parameter, regular physical activity can help mitigate depressive symptoms and fatigue (28).

9.7 SPINAL CORD INJURIES

In the area of spinal cord injuries, increased physical activity can play a number of important roles. Spinal cord injuries (SCI) can have enormous adverse initial effects on individuals and their family (29). SCI can force individuals and their families to cope with the effects of partial or complete paralysis of body movement and may also result in partial or complete loss of bodily functions such as sexual function and bowel and bladder control.

In the United States, there are about 12,000 new cases of SCI each year (30). There are about 260,000 individuals living with SCI. Regular physical activity can result in lowering the risk of co-morbidities, improving physical function, and improving health related quality of life. The types of activity that would be appropriate for individuals with SCI include arm ergometry for individuals with lower extremity paralysis, wheelchair-based exercise, underwater treadmills, and adapted forms of physical activity such as those where weight is partially supported.

Lowering the risk of CVD is particularly important in individuals with SCI since autonomic control of blood vessels may not be normal. Individuals with SCI carry 2–4 times the risk of CVD compared to those without SCI (31).

With regard to physical function, the effects of physical activity are significantly influenced by the location and severity of the injury. Some benefits from regular physical activity include reduction in shoulder pain (32), improvement of measures of vascular function, and possible improvements in physical fitness as well as improvement of wheel chair skills and propulsion for those who are wheelchair bound (33). Some benefits in physical function may improve walking for those who are able walk, improved upper extremity function and improved postural stability both in sitting and standing. Improvements in health related quality of life have also been demonstrated as well as a greater participation of physical activity and perceptions of quality of life.

9.8   PHYSICAL ACTIVITY AND INTELLECTUAL DISABILITIES

A wide spectrum of intellectual disabilities exists. Physical activity can play an important role in improving many of these conditions. For example, for Downs Syndrome, given advances in treatment, the median lifespan has risen from 25 years in 1983 to the current median of 60 years of age (34). Thus, individuals with Downs Syndrome are increasingly exposed to all of the comorbidities associated with aging and can benefit from increased physical activity in similar ways to individuals who do not have intellectual disabilities. For example, increased physical activity is likely to reduce the risk comorbid conditions such as cardiovascular disease in individuals with Downs Syndrome.

In addition, physical activity improves both physical function in both children and adults with intellectual disabilities. Downs Syndrome, which is the most common genetic cause of intellectual disability, has more than 250,000 individuals in the United States affected with the prevalence rising because of the increased lifespan in individuals with this condition (34).

In addition, increased physical activity has been demonstrated to improve health related quality of life in individuals with a diverse set of intellectual disabilities. All of these findings are particularly relevant given that currently 70% of adults with intellectual disabilities do not engage in health and wellness programs (35). The benefits for individuals with intellectual disabilities are also highly relevant to the aging process, including the increased prevalence of Alzheimer's disease in the elderly population. More information about the relationship between physical activity and intellectual disabilities may be found in Chapter 11.

9.9   CONCLUSIONS

Various disabilities and chronic conditions are very common in the US population. It has been estimated that over half of Americans have at least one chronic condition and about one third have multiple chronic conditions. The most common chronic conditions increase in prevalence with age. About 80% of adults over the age of 65 have multiple chronic conditions.

Physical activity has been shown to yield multiple health benefits for individuals with a variety of chronic conditions including cancer survivors, individuals with osteoarthritis, individuals with hypertension, individuals with T2DM, multiple sclerosis, spinal cord injury, and intellectual disabilities. While physical activity may yield benefits for other types of chronic conditions, these are the most prevalent.

The types of benefits that accrue from physical activity in individuals with chronic conditions include decreased risk of comorbid conditions, improvements in physical function, improvements in health related quality of life, and helping to mitigate disease progression. For all these reasons, individuals with chronic conditions should be counseled to increase their physical activity levels taking into account the specific type of chronic condition or conditions that they have.

CLINICAL APPLICATIONS

- Over half of individuals in the United States have at least one chronic condition.
- Increased physical activity has been shown to yield multiple benefits for individuals with a wide variety of chronic conditions.
- Physicians and other healthcare workers should assess the proper levels and types of physical activity for all individuals who have chronic conditions.
- Good data exist to suggest that increased physical activity yields important benefits to cancer survivors, osteoarthritis, hypertension, type 2 diabetes, multiple sclerosis, spinal cord injury, and intellectual disabilities. These constitute the most prevalent of the chronic conditions in the US population.

REFERENCES

1. Physical Activity Guidelines Advisory Committee. 2018 Physical Activity Guidelines Advisory Committee. 2018 Scientific Report. Individuals with Chronic Conditions. Washington, DC: U.S. Department of Health and Human Services.
2. U.S. Department of Health and Human Services. Multiple chronic conditions initiative. 2016. https://www.hhs.gov/ash/about-ash/multiple-chronic-conditions/about-mcc/index.html#_edn3 [Accessed January 24, 2020].
3. Gerteis J, Izrael D, Deitz D, et al. Multiple Chronic Conditions Chartbook. AHRQ Publications No, Q14- 0038. Agency for Healthcare Research and Quality (Rockville, MD); April 2014.
4. Physical Activity Guidelines Advisory Committee. Physical Activity Guidelines Advisory Committee Report, 2008. Washington, DC: US Department of Health and Human Services; 2008. https://health.gov/paguidelines/guidelines/report.aspx. Published 2008 [Accessed January 24, 2020].
5. National Cancer Institute; Surveillance, Epidemiology, and End Results Program. Cancer stat facts: cancer of any site. https://seer.cancer.gov/statfacts/html/all.html [Accessed January 24, 2020].
6. National Cancer Institute; Surveillance, Epidemiology, and End Results Program. Cancer stat facts: female breast cancer. https://seer.cancer.gov/statfacts/html/breast.html [Accessed January 24, 2020].
7. National Cancer Institute; Surveillance, Epidemiology, and End Results Program. Cancer stat facts: colorectal cancer. https://seer.cancer.gov/statfacts/html/colorect.html [Accessed January 24, 2020].

8. American Cancer Society. Key statistics for colorectal cancer. https://www.cancer.org/content/dam/CRC/PDF/Public/8604.00.pdf [Accessed January 24, 2020].

9. National Cancer Institute; Surveillance, Epidemiology, and End Results Program. Cancer stat facts: prostate cancer. https://seer.cancer.gov/statfacts/html/prost.html [Accessed January 24, 2020].

10. National Cancer Institute. SEER Cancer Statistics Review 1975–2012, table 12. https://seer.cancer.gov/archive/csr/1975_2012/browse_csr.php?sectionSEL=2&pageSEL=sect_02_table.12 [Accessed January 24, 2020].

11. National Cancer Institute. SEER Cancer Statistics Review 1975–2012, table 9. https://seer.cancer.gov/archive/csr/1975_2012/browse_csr.php?sectionSEL=2&pageSEL=sect_02_table.09 [Accessed January 24, 2020].

12. Cisternas MG, Murphy L, Sacks JJ, et al. Alternative methods for defining osteoarthritis and the impact on estimating prevalence in a U.S. Population-based survey. Arthritis Care Res (Hoboken). 2016;68(5):574–580. doi:10.1002/acr.22721.

13. Cross M, Smith E, Hoy D, et al. The global burden of hip and knee osteoarthritis: estimates from the global burden of disease 2010 study. Ann Rheum Dis. 2014;73(7):1323–1330. doi:10.1136/annrheumdis2013-204763.

14. Deshpande BR, Katz JN, Solomon DH, et al. Number of persons with symptomatic knee osteoarthritis in the US: impact of race and ethnicity, age, sex, and obesity. Arthritis Care Res (Hoboken). 2016;68(12):1743–1750. doi:10.1002/acr.22897.

15. Hootman JM, Helmick CG, Barbour KE, et al. Updated projected prevalence of selfreported doctor-diagnosed arthritis and arthritis-attributable activity limitation among U.S. Adults, 2015- 2040. Arthritis Rheumatol. 2016;68(7):1582–1587. doi:10.1002/art.39692.

16. Chobanian AV, Bakris GL, Black HR, et al. Seventh report of the joint national committee on prevention, detection, evaluation, and treatment of High blood pressure. Hypertension. 2003;42(6):1206–1252.

17. Whelton PK, Carey RM, Aronow WS, et al. 2017 acc/aha/aapa/abc/acpm/ags/apha/ash/aspc/nma/pcna guideline for the prevention, detection, evaluation, and management of high blood pressure in adults: a report of the american college of cardiology/american heart association task force on clinical practice guidelines. J Am Coll Cardiol. 2018;71:e127–e248

18. Cornelissen VA, Smart NA. Exercise training for blood pressure: a systematic review and meta-analysis. J Am Heart Assoc. 2013;2(1):e004473. doi:10.1161/JAHA.112.004473. 10.1161/JAHA.112.004473.

19. Centers for Disease Control and Prevention. National Diabetes Statistics Report, 2017. https://www.cdc.gov/diabetes/pdfs/data/statistics/national-diabetes-statistics-report.pdf [Accessed January 24, 2020].

20. Kodama S, Tanaka S, Heianza Y, et al. Association between physical activity and risk of all-cause mortality and cardiovascular disease in patients with diabetes: a meta-analysis. Diabetes Care. 2013;36(2):471–479. doi:10.2337/dc12-0783.

21. Centers for Disease Control and Prevention. Diabetes quick facts. https://www.cdc.gov/diabetes/basics/quick-facts.html [Accessed January 24, 2020].

22. American Diabetes Association. Lifestyle management. Sec. 4. In Standards of Medical Care in Diabetes–2017. Diabetes Care. 2017;40(suppl 1):S33–S43.

23. Sadarangani KP, Hamer M, Mindell JS, et al. Physical activity and risk of all-cause and cardiovascular disease mortality in diabetic adults from Great Britain: pooled analysis of 10 population-based cohorts. Diabetes Care. 2014;37(4):1016–1023. doi:10.2337/dc13-1816.

24. The Diabetes Prevention Program Research G. The diabetes prevention program (dpp): description of lifestyle intervention *Diabetes Care.* 2002;25:2165–2171.

25. Dietz WH, Robinson TN. Clinical practice. Overweight children and adolescents N Engl J Med. 2005;352:2100–2109.

26. Latimer-Cheung AE, Pilutti AE, Hicks AL, et al. Effects of exercise training on fitness, mobility, fatigue, and health-related quality of life among adults with multiple sclerosis: a systematic review to inform guideline development. Arch Phys Med Rehabil. 2013;94(9):1800–1828.e3. doi:10.1016/j.apmr.2013.04.020.

27. Ensari I, Motl RW, Pilutti LA. Exercise training improves depressive symptoms in people with multiple sclerosis: results of a meta-analysis. J Psychosom Res. 2014;76(6):465–471. doi:10.1016/j.jpsychores.2014.03.014.

28. Dalgas U, Stenager E, Sloth M, Stenager E. The effect of exercise on depressive symptoms in multiple sclerosis based on a meta-analysis and critical review of the literature. Eur J Neurol. 2015;22(3):443–e34. doi:10.1111/ene.12576

29. Brainandspinalcord.org. Spinal cord injury statistics. https://www.brainandspinalcord.org/spinal-cord-injury-statistics/ [Accessed January 24, 2020].

30. Myers J, Lee M, Kiratli J. Cardiovascular disease in spinal cord injury: an overview of prevalence, risk, evaluation, and management. Am J Phys Med Rehabil. 2007;86(2):142–152. doi:10.1097/PHM.0b013e31802f0247

31. Cragg JJ, Noonan VK, Krassioukov A, et al. Cardiovascular disease and spinal cord injury: results from a national population health survey. Neurology. 2013;81(8):723–728. doi:10.1212/WNL.0b013e3182a1aa68.

32. Jain NB, Higgins LD, Katz JN, et al. Association of shoulder pain with the use of mobility devices in persons with chronic spinal cord injury. PMR. 2010;2(10):896–900. doi:10.1016/j.pmrj.2010.05.004.

33. Cratsenberg KA, Deitrick CE, Harrington TK, et al. Effectiveness of exercise programs for management of shoulder pain in manual wheelchair users with spinal cord injury. J Neurol Phys Ther. 2015;39(4):197–203. doi:10.1097/NPT.0000000000000103.

34. Presson AP, Partyka G, Jensen KM, et al. Current estimate of Down syndrome population prevalence in the United States. J Pediatr. 2013;163(4):1163–1168. doi:10.1016/j.jpeds.2013.06.013.

35. Office of Disease Prevention and Health Promotion. 2020 topics and objectives: disability and health. https://www.healthypeople.gov/2020/topics-objectives/topic/disability-and-health [Accessed January 24, 2020].

10 Physical Activity, Weight Gain, and Obesity

KEY POINTS

- Overweight and obesity are significant public health issues in the US affecting approximately 70% of the adult population.
- Physical activity is a powerful modality for lowering the risk of weight gain.
- Physical activity by itself conveys only modest benefits in initial weight loss.
- A combination of physical activity and energy restriction together are key modalities in weight loss.
- Physical activity plays a very important role in long-term maintenance of weight loss.
- Increased physical activity lowers risk factors for various chronic diseases associated with obesity independent of weight loss.

10.1 WEIGHT GAIN AND PHYSICAL ACTIVITY

Weight gain and lack of physical activity are both independently associated with increased risk of cardiovascular disease (CVD), type 2 diabetes (T2DM), and the Metabolic Syndrome (METS) (1–7). Recent estimates indicate that the prevalence of overweight (body mass index (BMI) 25–30 kg/m^2) in the United States for adult men is approximately 40% and for women is 30% (8). Estimates for obesity (BMI ≥30 kg/m^2) for men are approximately 35% and for women approximately 40%. Thus, the prevalence of overweight or obesity amongst adults in the United States is approximately 70%.

There is an urgent need to discover and deliver effective treatments for both overweight and obesity. Furthermore, strategies to prevent or minimize weight gain which may contribute to lowering the prevalence of overweight and obesity are also very important (9–15). Physical activity plays multiple roles both in the reduction of the risk of weight gain and in the treatment of both overweight and obesity (16–20).

Overweight and obesity are both associated with increased risk of CVD and particularly T2DM which comprises 90–95% of all diabetes (21). Physical activity is an important lifestyle modality which has been utilized for both prevention and treatment of obesity, CVD, and T2DM. Physical activity plays a key role in all of these conditions. (See also Chapters 3 and 5.)

10.2 THE EFFECTS OF PHYSICAL ACTIVITY ON PREVENTION OF WEIGHT GAIN

The Physical Activity Guidelines Advisory 2018 Scientific Report (2018 PAGA) has rated the evidence for the relationship of greater amounts of physical activity and decreased weight gain in adults as "strong" (22). The PAGA 2018 also reported that evidence indicates that the relationship is more pronounced if physical activity exposure exceeds 150 minutes per week.

From a public health perspective, it is important to not only consider the role of effective treatments for weight loss but also approaches to prevent weight gain. There are multiple, cross-sectional studies to support an inverse relationship between physical activity and both body mass index and body fatness. Prospective data also exists from the Women's Health Study (18), the National Health and Nutrition Examination Survey-1 (NHANES-1) Epidemiologic Follow-up Study (14), the Harvard Alumni Study (19), and the Aerobic Center Longitudinal Research Study (17) to support the importance of physical activity in the prevention of weight gain.

Other studies have demonstrated that physical activity is important for maintaining a healthy body weight (BMI 19 $\leq$25 kg/m^2) and also reducing the likelihood of developing obesity (911). It appears that the threshold for physical activity needed to prevent significant weight gain (defined as an increase of at least 3% body weight) is between 150–250 minutes per week (23).

10.3   EFFECT OF PHYSICAL ACTIVITY ON WEIGHT LOSS

10.3.1   REGULAR AEROBIC ACTIVITY

Regular aerobic physical activity is a key intervention recommended by a variety of organizations as a component of treatment of overweight and obesity. The role of physical activity in weight loss, however, without concurrent reduction of energy intake, appears to be modest. In one study, for example, where overweight adults were prescribed home-based physical activity without concurrent reduction in energy intake, the weight loss was only 2% at six months and 1% at 18 months (24). Other studies have corroborated these findings (25, 26). These findings are consistent with the findings reported in the Physical Activity Guidelines Advisory Committee Report of 2008 and PAGA 2018. The position statement from the American College of Sports Medicine (ACSM) in 2009 reported that there was no significant change in body weight in response to less than 150 minutes per week of physical activity. In one study, physical activity of greater than 150 and 225–420 minutes per week resulted in weight loss between 2.3 kg and 5.75 kg respectively (24).

10.3.2   RESISTANCE EXERCISE

Relatively few studies exist specifically on the effect of resistance exercise on weight loss. It has been postulated that resistance exercise during weight loss may be beneficial because of its potential role in increasing lean mass. This could result in increased resting metabolic rate and also increased strength. These benefits may result in increased free living physical activity in addition to the energy expenditure from resistance exercise itself (27–31). It has also been reported that resistance exercise may reduce subcutaneous abdominal adiposity (32). Thus, the benefits of resistance exercise for individuals with obesity may result from improvements in lean mass and strength, and reductions in abdominal adiposity rather than reductions in total body fat.

10.3.3 WALKING

Walking represents a convenient way of increasing physical activity and is often included both in programs for weight loss or to prevent weight gain (33–36). Several studies have shown that individuals who accumulate more than 10,000 walking steps at least three times per week may get benefits related to weight loss (37). One study showed that a combination of walking and resistance strength training resulted in more weight loss benefits than either modality alone.

10.3.4 LIFESTYLE ACTIVITIES

Structured forms of physical activity may result in increases in energy expenditure and can play an important role in interventions for weight loss. A number of these studies have utilized pedometers to encourage individuals to increase their level of physical activity. Several studies have shown that individuals who increase their steps from 2,100 to 3,000 steps per day have lost between 2 and 3 kilograms of body weight (38). There does not appear to be any difference between supervised or unsupervised structure with regard to step count. However, there may be additional benefits for maintenance of weight loss for individuals who accumulate more than 10,000 steps per day.

10.3.5 SEDENTARY BEHAVIOR

The PAGA 2018 Scientific Report concluded there was "limited" evidence of a relationship between the amount of time spent in sedentary behavior and higher levels of adiposity. Several studies, however, have shown that if sedentary behavior is substituted by increased physical activity, such as walking, this may represent an effective strategy for increasing energy expenditure and result in weight loss (39).

10.3.6 DURATION OF PHYSICAL ACTIVITY BOUTS

A number of studies previously reported that physical activity bouts of at least 8–10 minutes per session were required in order to be an effective component of weight loss (40). However, the PAGA 2018 Scientific Report, cited evidence from cross-sectional studies that even bouts of physical activity of less than 10 minutes may result in a lower body mass index and body fatness when combined with energy restriction. Some studies, however, have suggested activity bouts of greater than 10 minutes are required (41). Thus, the issue of duration of physical activity bouts as part of a weight loss program remains in question.

10.3.7 COMBINATION OF AEROBIC PHYSICAL ACTIVITY AND ENERGY RESTRICTION

The standard recommendation for weight loss is to combine physical activity with a reduction in energy intake (7). A number of studies have shown that physical activity, when added to energy restriction, can achieve weight loss beyond what energy restriction alone is capable of doing. One study by Goodpaster and colleagues reported that the addition of physical activity to energy restriction increased weight loss at 6 months by 2.7 kilograms (42). A second study by Wing et al demonstrated similar findings with a combined treatment resulting in an increase of 1.2 kilograms in weight loss (26).

10.3.8 LONG-TERM BENEFITS OF PHYSICAL ACTIVITY FOR WEIGHT LOSS

Physical activity may also be important for enhancing weight loss beyond the initial six months of treatment and improve the long-term maintenance of weight loss while minimizing the weight regain. Results of a 24-month study by Jacicic et al. in overweight and obese women increased physical activity by 1,500 kcals per week and achieved a weight loss of 14.2 kilograms (16.8% of initial body weight) (43–45), while less weight loss was observed in 24 months of lower levels of physical activity (46). These findings suggest that relatively high levels of physical activity may be necessary to improve long-term weight loss. To put this in perspective, 1,500 kcals per week is the equivalent of approximately an additional 275 minutes per week of brisk walking above normal baseline levels (47). Other studies have shown similar findings. It may also be necessary for this physical activity to occur in bouts of at least 10 minutes. Several studies by Jacicic et al. have supported this finding with an accumulation of 200–300 minutes per week associated with improved weight loss at eighteen months in the context of a combination of physical activity and energy restriction (48).

10.4 THE ROLE OF PHYSICAL ACTIVITY IN SURGICALLY INDUCED WEIGHT LOSS

Bariatric surgery has become an increasingly common and effective treatment for weight loss, particularly for individuals with high levels of obesity and/or obesity with other risk factors for cardiovascular disease and diabetes. Preliminary data have suggested that greater weight loss occurs in bariatric surgical patients who participate in greater than 150 minutes per week in physical activity compared to patients participating in less than 150 minutes per week (49). Furthermore, other research has shown that improvements in weight loss at 6 and 24 months occur following bariatric surgery if these levels of physical activity are included in the postoperative treatment (49–50). Unfortunately, few patients following bariatric surgery meet these guidelines to experience these benefits (51). It is important to consider the psychological and social support needed in the postoperative period in order to increase the likelihood of physical activity following bariatric surgery.

10.5 WEIGHT LOSS VARIABILITY IN RESPONSE TO PHYSICAL ACTIVITY

There is considerable variability in weight loss in response to physical activity. In one study the weight loss in response to four months of controlled exercise resulted in a range of weight loss equivalent to approximately 3–12 kilograms (53). The exact cause of this high level of variability is not known. It is, however, important to factor this variability into the physical activity prescription following weight loss.

One component of this variability may be a cluster of biological factors. In one study of twins examined over a period of 93 days, weight loss in response to physical activity was similar in each pair of twins, but highly variable between pairs of twins (54). The exact biological factors at play have yet to be determined.

10.6 IMPACTS OF PHYSICAL ACTIVITY ON OTHER COMPONENTS OF ENERGY EXPENDITURE

Physical activity is an important and variable component of total energy expenditure that may exert a significant influence on the ability to create a negative energy balance (55). There appears to be an acute increase in resting metabolic rate (RMR) in response to physical activity. Regular physical activity participation may also be associated with higher, long-term RMR (56). It should be noted, however, that weight loss causes a decrease in RMR (57), particularly with significant weight loss. Thus, physical activity may counterbalance decreases in RMR during and following weight loss.

10.7 INFLUENCE OF PHYSICAL ACTIVITY ON ENERGY INTAKE

The response of energy intake to physical activity is quite variable. One study reported an increase in negative energy balance in response to 50 minutes of physical activity (58). Another study, however, reported that a majority of patients consumed more calories following 35–45 minutes of physical activity compared to a seated rest period (59). Thus, in some patients it appears that physical activity increases hunger and appetite, whereas in others it may enhance satiety.

10.8 FACTORS INFLUENCING ADHERENCE TO PHYSICAL ACTIVITY

In many instances, individuals who are overweight or obese may have difficulty changing behavior to become more physically active. Behavior change and adherence to new behaviors is difficult for all people, but may be particularly difficult for individuals who have been inactive in their lives or who are overweight or obese. Self-efficacy has been demonstrated in a few studies to influence whether or not overweight or obese people are able to stick with exercise programs (60). Some literature also suggests that there may be genetic factors at play. All of these factors suggest that individuals who are prescribing increased physical activity need specific training in behavior change when treating overweight or obese adults and recommending physical activity as a component of the intervention plan.

10.9 PHYSICAL ACTIVITY, FITNESS, AND HEALTH OUTCOMES

A number of studies have shown that cardiorespiratory fitness improves in overweight or obese individuals when physical activity is included as a component of an intervention program. These benefits are present whether or not the intervention results in weight loss (61). In contrast, cardiorespiratory fitness does not improve simply through energy restriction (62, 63). Thus, physical activity is a very significant component in intervention for overweight and obese adults that results in improved cardiorespiratory fitness.

The magnitude of improvement in fitness depends on the dose of physical activity performed as it does in healthy weight individuals. Importantly, the level of cardiorespiratory fitness is strongly associated with reduction in risk of various chronic diseases, such as CVD and T2DM. In addition, the benefit of physical activity on fitness in overweight and obese adults provides another reason for recommending physical activity as a component of weight loss or prevention of weight gain in overweight and obese individuals.

These findings have been documented in a number of studies and have been classified as components of the "fitness versus fatness" debate (64–66). Higher levels of fitness are an important factor in reducing the risk of mortality, independent of the influence of body fatness. It should be emphasized, however, that most data do not support the concept that increased fitness in overweight or obese individuals totally reverses the risk of the high level of BMI or body fatness.

Data from the Lipid Research Clinic Study suggest that both fitness and fatness contribute to risk for mortality (67). In the Look AHEAD Study individuals with T2DM who achieved a weight loss of at least 10% over the first year of treatment and significantly increased physical activity which resulted in a 20% reduction in the primary outcome of CVD (composite of death from CVD, non- fatal acute myocardial infarction, nonfatal stroke, and hospital admission for angina) (68). These findings underscore the importance that interventions for overweight and obese adults should focus on both weight loss and improving fitness to reduce the risk of both all cause and cardiovascular disease mortality.

10.10   EFFECTS ON RISK FACTORS FOR CARDIOVASCULAR DISEASE

Obesity in and of itself is a significant risk factor for CVD. In addition, obesity interacts with other risk factors for CVD including blood pressure, lipids, and diabetes. Physical activity may play a role in lowering the risk of cardiovascular disease in overweight and obese individuals, as it does in healthy weight individuals (see also Chapter 3).

A number of studies have shown that overweight and obesity are associated with the risk of developing hypertension. A study by Rankin et al. demonstrated that cardiorespiratory fitness attenuates that risk (69). Chen et al. reported that BMI had a closer relationship to systolic blood pressure than did fitness (70). Wing et al. reported that both BMI and cardiorespiratory fitness were significantly associated with systolic blood pressure in women whether or not they were taking medicine for blood pressure control (71). In men not taking medication for blood pressure control, however, BMI and fitness were not associated with systolic blood pressure. These findings suggest that both BMI and fitness are important for blood pressure control in overweight and obese adults.

Overweight and obesity are also associated with abnormal lipid patterns. Physical activity appears to play a modest role in controlling cholesterol. Weight loss typically lowers total cholesterol by 3–4 mg/dL. Low-density lipoproteins (LDL) were reduced by 3.0 mg/dL in one study in response to a physical activity intervention (72). Physical activity interventions and fitness also have been repeatedly shown to increase high-density lipoprotein-c (HDL-C) (72). These findings suggest that both body fatness and physical activity can play roles in lipid reduction in overweight and obese individuals.

It is well known that excess adiposity increases markers of inflammation such as C-reactive protein (CRP), Interleukin-6 (IL6) tissue necrosis factor α (TNFα) as well as the antithrombotic factor adiponectin (73). Inflammation plays a key role in the development of atherosclerosis. Nonetheless, several other studies have not demonstrated that increased physical activity by itself in individuals with overweight or obesity lowers anti-inflammatory response (74, 75).

10.11   CONCLUSIONS

Physical activity, as outlined in multiple chapters in this book, contributes to numerous health benefits. Physical activity also plays a very significant role in the management of body weight, particularly in the prevention of weight gain and as an adjunct in therapy for overweight or obesity.

CLINICAL APPLICATIONS

- Physical activity should be a component of weight loss in all individuals who are overweight or obese.
- Physical activity plays an important role in reducing the likelihood of weight gain and should be prescribed to individuals who are normal weight, overweight or obese.
- Physical activity may play a role in lowering the risk of high blood pressure in overweight or obese individuals.
- Physical activity is an important component of long-term maintenance of weight loss.
- All clinicians should assess and discuss the importance of physical activity in every clinical encounter with overweight or obese individuals.

REFERENCES

1. Rippe J, Angelopoulos T. Obesity and health. In Rippe JM. Lifestyle Medicine (2nd edition). CRC Press (Boca Raton, FL), 2013.
2. Rippe J, Angelopoulos T. Obesity and heart disease. In Rippe JM and Angelopoulos TA (eds). Obesity: Prevention and Treatment. CRC Press (Boca Raton, FL), 2012.
3. Rippe J, Angelopoulos T. Preventing and managing obesity: The scope of the problem. In Rippe JM and Angelopoulos TA (eds). Obesity: Prevention and Treatment. CRC Press (Boca Raton, FL), 2012.
4. Jakicic J, Rogers R, Collins K. Exercise management for the obese patient. In Rippe JM. Lifestyle Medicine (3rd edition). CRC Press (Boca Raton), 2019.
5. Flegal K, Kruszon-Moran D, Carroll M, et al. Trends in obesity among adults in the United States, 2005 to 2014. JAMA. 2016;315:2284–2291.

6. Jensen M, Ryan D, Apovian C, et al. 2013 AHA/ACC/TOS guideline for the management of overweight and obesity in adults: a report of the American College of Cardiology/American heart association task force on practice guidelines and the obesity society. J Am Coll Cardiol. 2014;63:2985–3023.
7. National Institutes of Health National Heart Lung and Blood Institute. Clinical guidelines on the identification, evaluation, and treatment of overweight and obesity in adults - the evidence report. Obes Res. 1998;6(suppl.2).
8. National Center for Health Statistics Health, United States, 2016: With Chartbook on Long-Term Trends in Healthy. Hyattsville, MD, 2017.
9. Cameron N, Nichols J, Hill L, et al. Associations betweeen physical activity and BMI, body fatness, and visceral adiposity in overweight or obese latino and non-latino adults. Int J Obes. 2017;41:873–877.
10. Fan J, Brown B, Hanson H, et al. Moderate to vigorous physical activity and weight outcomes: does every minute count? Am J Prev Med. 2013;28:41–49.
11. Glazer N, Lyass A, Esliger D, et al. Sustained and shorter bouts of physical activity are related to cardiovascular health. Med Sci Sports Exerc. 2013;45:109–115.
12. Jakicic J, Gregg E, Knowler W, et al. Physical activity patterns of overweight and obese individuals with type 2 diabetes in the look AHEAD study. Med Sci Sports Exerc. 2010;42:1995–2005.
13. Jefferis B, Parsons T, Sartini C, et al. Does duration of physical activity bouts matter for adiposity and metabolic syndrome? A cross-sectional study of older British men. Int J Behav Nutr Phys Act. 2016;13.
14. Loprinzi P, Cardinal B. Association between biologic outcomes and objectively measured physical activity accumulated in >10-minute bout and <10-minute bouts Am J Health Promot. 2013;27:143–151.
15. Wolff-Hughes D, Fitzhugh E, Bassett D, et al. Total activity counts and bouted minutes of moderate-to-vigorous physical activity: relationships with cardiometabolic biomarkers using 2003-2006 NHANES. J Phys Act Health. 2015;12:694–700.
16. Williamson D, Madans J, Anda R, et al. Recreational physical activity and ten-year weight change in a US national cohort. Int J Obes. 1993;17:279–286.
17. DiPietro L, Dziura J, Blair S. Estimated change in physical activity level (PAL) and prediction of 5-year weight change in men: the aerobics center longitudinal study Int J Obes. 2004;28:1541–1547.
18. Lee I, Djousse L, Sesso H, et al. Physical activity and weight gain prevention. JAMA. 2010;303:1173–1179.
19. Shiroma E, Sesso H, Lee I. Physical activity and weight gain prevention in older men. Int J Obes (Lond). 2012;36:1165–1169.
20. Brown W, Kabir E, Clark B, et al. Maintaining a healthy BMI. Data from a 16-year study of young Australian women. Am J Prev Med. 2016;51:e165–e178.
21. Colberg S, Sigal R, Yardley J, et al. Physical Activity/Exercise and diabetes: a position statement of the American diabetes association. Diabetes Care. 2016;39:2065–2079.
22. 2018 Physical Activity Guidelines Advisory Committee. 2018 Physical Activity Guidelines Advisory Committee Scientific Report. Washington, DC: U.S. Department of Health and Human Services, 2018.
23. Donnelly J, Blair S, Jakicic J, et al. ACSM position stand on appropriate intervention strategies for weight loss and prevention of weight regain for adults. Med Sci Sports Exerc. 2009;42:459–471.
24. Jakicic J, Otto A, Semler L, et al. Effect of physical activity on 18-month weight change in overweight adults. Obesity. 2011;19:100–109.
25. Hagan R, Upton S, Wong L, et al. The effects of aerobic conditioning and/or calorie restriction in overweight men and women. Med Sci Sports Exerc. 1986;18:87–94.

26. Wing R, Venditti E, Jakicic J, et al. Lifestyle intervention in overweight individuals with a family history of diabetes. Diabetes Care. 1998;21:350–359.
27. Donnelly J, Jakicic J, Pronk N, et al. Is resistance exercise effective for weight management? Evid Based Prevent Med. 2004;1:21–29.
28. Hunter G, Bryan D, Wetzstein C, et al. Reistance training and intra-abdominal adipose tissue in older men and women. Med Sci Sports Exerc. 2002;34:1023–1028.
29. Hunter G, Wetzstein C, Fields D, et al. Resistance training increases total energy expenditure and free-living physical activity in older adults. J Appl Physiol. 2000;89:977–984.
30. Olson T, Dengel D, Leon A, et al. Changes in inflammatory biomarkers following one-year of moderate resistance exercise in overweight women. Int J Obesity. 2007;31:996–1003.
31. Schmitz K, Jensen M, Kugler K, et al. Strength training for obesity prevention in midlife women. Int J Obes Relat Meta Disord. 2003;27:326–333.
32. Janssen I, Ross R. Effects of sex on the change in visceral, subcutaneous adipose tissue and skeletal muscle in response to weight loss. Int J Obes Relat Meta Disord. 1999;23:1035–1046.
33. Kashiwa A, Rippe JM. Fitness Walking for Women. Putnam (N.Y.), 1987.
34. Rippe J, Ward A, Porcari J, Freedson PS. Walking for health and fitness. JAMA. 1988;259:272.
35. Rockport 1-Mile Fitness Walking Test Calculator. https://www.verywellfit.com/rockport-fitness-walking-test-calculator-395269636.
36. Rippe J, Ward A. The Complete Book of Fitness Walking. Prentice Hall Press (New York), 1990.
37. Creasy S, Rogers R, Gibbs B, et al. Effects of supervised and unsupervised physical activity programmes for weight loss. Obesity Sci Pract. 2017;3: 143–152.
38. Chan C, Ryan D, Tudor-Locke C. Health benefits of a pedometer-based physical activity intervention in sedentary workers. Prev Med. 2004;39:1215–1222.
39. Creasy S, Rogers R, Byard T, et al. Energy expenditure during acute periods of sitting, standing, and walking. J Phys Act Health. 2016;13:573–578.
40. Pate R, Pratt M, Blair S, et al. Physical activity and public health: a recommendation from the centers for disease and prevention and the American College of sports medicine. JAMA. 1995;273:402–407.
41. White D, Pettee G, Kim Y, et al. Do short spurts of physical activity benefit health? The CARDIA study. Med Sci Sports Exerc. 2015;47:2353–2358.
42. Goodpaster B, DeLany J, Otto A, et al. Effects of diet and physical activity interventions on weight loss and cardiometabolic risk factors in severely obese adults: a randomized trial. JAMA. 2010;304:1795–1802.
43. Jeffery R, Wing R, Sherwood N, et al. Physical activity and weight loss: does prescribing higher physical activity goals improve outcome? Am J Clin Nutr. 2003;78: 684–689.
44. Klem M, Wing R, McGuire MT, et al. A descriptive study of individuals successful at long-term maintenance of substantial weight loss. Am J Clin Nutr. 1997;66:239–246.
45. Schoeller D, Shay K, Kushner R. How much physical activity is needed to minimize weight gain in previously obese women? Am J Clin Nutr. 1997;66:551–556.
46. Jakicic J, Marcus B, Lang W, et al. Effect of exercise on 24-month weight loss in overweight women. Arch Int Med. 2008;168:1550–1559.
47. Unick J, Jakicic J, Marcus B. Contribution of behavior intervention components to 24 month weight loss. Med Sci Sports Exerc. 2010;42:745–753.
48. Jakicic J, Tate D, Lang W, et al. Objective physical activity and weight loss in adults: the step-Up randomized clinical trial. Obesity. 2014;22:2284–2292.
49. Evans R, Bond D, Wolfe L, et al. Participation in 150 minutes/week of moderate or higher intensity physical activity yields greater weight loss following gastric bypass surgery. Surg Obes Relat Dis. 2007;3:526–530.

50. Bond D, Evans R, Wolfe L, et al. Impact of self-reported physical activity participation on proportion of excess weight loss and BMI among gastric bypass surgery patients. The American Surgeon. 2004;70:811–814.

51. Bergh I, Kvalem I, Mala T, et al. Predictors of physical activity after gastric bypass - a prospective study. Obes Surg. 2017;27:2050–2057.

52. Josbeno D, Kalarchian M, Sparto P, et al. Physical activity and physical function in individuals post-bariatric surgery. Obes Surg. 2011;21:1243–1249.

53. Bouchard C, Tremblay A, Nadeau A, et al. Long-term exercise training and constant energy intake. 1: effect on body composition and selected metabolic variables. Int J Obesity. 1990;14:57–73.

54. Bouchard C, Tremblay A, Despres J, et al. The response to exercise with constant energy intake in identical twins. Obesity Res. 1994;2:400–410.

55. Ravussin E, Bogardus C. Relationship of genetics, age, and physical fitness to daily energy expenditure and fuel utilization. Am J Clin Nutr. 1989;49:968–975.

56. Tremblay A, Fontaine E, Poehlman E, et al. The effect of exercise-training on resting metabolic rate in lean and moderately obese individuals. Int J Obesity. 1986;10:511–517.

57. Tremblay A. Physical activity level and resting metabolic rate. In: Bouchard C, Katzmarzyk PT (eds). Physical Activity and Obesity (2nd edition). Human Kinetics (Chamaign, IL), 2010.

58. Finlayson G, Bryant E, Blundell J, et al. Acute compensatory eating following exercise is associated with implicit hedonic wanting for food. Physiol Behav. 2009;97: 62–67.

59. Unick J, Otto A, Helsel D, et al. The acute effect of exercise on energy intake in overweight/obese women. Appetite. 2010;55:413–419.

60. Gallagher K, Jakicic J, Napolitano M, et al. Psychosocial factors related to physical activity and weight loss in overweight women. Med Sci Sports Exerc. 2006;38:971–980.

61. Ross R, Dagnone D, Jones P, et al. Reduction in obesity and related comorbid conditions after diet-induced weight loss or exercise-induced weight loss in men. Ann Intern Med. 2000;133:92–103.

62. Donnelly J, Pronk N, Jacobsen D, et al. Effects of a very-low-calorie diet and physical-training regimenson body composition and resting metabolic rate in obese females. Am J Clin Nutr. 1991;54:56–61.

63. Church T, Earnest C, Skinner J, et al. Effects of different doses of physical activity on cardiorespiratory fitness among sedentary, overweight or obese postmenopausal women with elevated blood pressure. JAMA. 2007;297:2081–2091.

64. Blair S, Kohl H, Paffenbarger R, et al. Physical fitness and all-cause mortality. A prospective study of healthy men and women. JAMA. 1989;262:2395–2401.

65. Barlow C, Kohl H, Gibbons L, et al. Physical activity, mortality, and obesity. Int J Obes. 1995;19:S41–S44.

66. Church T, LaMonte M, Barlow C, et al. Cardiorespiratory fitness and body mass index as predictors of cardiovascular disease mortality among men with diabetes. Arch Intern Med. 2005;165:2114–2120.

67. Stevens J, Cai J, Evenson K, et al. Fitness and fatness as predictors of mortality from all causes and from cardiovascular disease in men and women in the lipid research clinics study. Am J Epidemiol. 2002;156:832–841.

68. The Look AHEAD Research Group. Association of the magnitude of weight loss and changes in physical fitness with long-term cardiovascular disease outcomes in overweight or obese people with type 2 diabetes: a post-hoc analysis of the look AHEAD randomised clinical trial. Lancet Diabetes Endocrinol. 2016;4:913–921.

69. Rankinen T, Church T, Rice T, et al. Cardiorespiratory fitness, BMI, and risk of hypertension: the HYPGENE study. Med Sci Sports Exerc. 2007;39:1687–1692.

70. Chen J, Das S, Barlow C, et al. Fitness, fatness, and systolic blood pressure: data from the cooper center longitudinal study. Am Heart J. 2010;160:166–170.

71. Wing R, Jakicic J, Neiberg R, et al. Fitness, fatness, and cardiovascular risk factors in type 2 diabetes: look AHEAD study. Med Sci Sports Exerc. 2007;39:2107–2116.

72. Kelley G, Kelley K, Tran Z. Aerobic exercise, lipids and lipoproteins in overweight and obese adults: a meta-analysis of randomized controlled trials. Int J Obes. 2005;29: 881–893.

73. Church T, Earnest C, Thompson A, et al. Exercise without weight loss does not reduce C-reactive protein: the INFLAME study. Med Sci Sports Exerc. 2010;42:708–716.

74. Nicklas B, Ambrosius W, Messier S, et al. Diet-induced weight loss, exercise, and chronic inflammation in older, obese adults: a randomized controlled clinical trial. Am J Clin Nutr. 2004;79:544–551.

75. Hamer M, Steptoe A. Prospective study of physical fitness, adiposity, and inflammatory markers in healthy middle-aged men and women. Am J Clin Nutr. 2009;89:85–89.

11 Physical Activity, Cognition, and Brain Health

KEY POINTS

- Physical activity is a key component of brain health throughout the lifespan.
- Physical activity enhances cognition throughout the lifespan.
- Physical activity decreases the likelihood of various dementias including Alzheimer's disease.
- Physical activity improves biomarkers of brain health.
- Physical activity plays an important role in enhancing affect and decreasing anxiety and tension.
- Physical activity plays an important role in all aspects of sleep.

11.1 INTRODUCTION

As the worldwide population continues to age, issues related to brain health have increasingly become important and entered the scientific literature. As used in this chapter, the same definition that was adopted by the Physical Activity Guidelines for Americans Advisory Committee 2018 Scientific Report (PAGA) will be used for brain health as a concept involving the "optimal or maximal functioning of behavioral and biological measures of the brain and its subjective experiences arising from the brain function" (e.g., mood) (1). There are multiple aspects of brain health that include cognition, reduction in the risk of dementia, perceptions of Quality of Life (QoL), and sleep. In addition, recent advances in technology have allowed measurement of variety of biological markers in the brain. With all of these factors in mind, it is a propitious time to consider issues related to brain health both from an individual and from a public health standpoint.

Numerous studies have shown that there is a strong and positive relationship between physical activity and brain health (2–16). This is one of the major reasons that the American Heart Association (AHA) and the American Stroke Association (ASA) joined forces to issue a Presidential Advisory on "Optimizing Brain Health" (17).

This chapter will explore a variety of domains that are now considered part of brain health particularly as they are related to the important role of physical activity in preserving brain health.

11.2   PHYSICAL ACTIVITY AND COGNITION

According to the PAGA 2018 Scientific Report, moderate evidence exists associating greater amounts of physical activity with improvements in cognition (3, 12–16). These include academic achievement, various tests involving processing speed, memory, and executive function as well as decreased risk of dementia. These effects have been found across a variety of forms of physical activity including aerobic activity (e.g., brisk walking), muscle strengthening, yoga, and play activities (e.g., tag or other simple-rule organization games).

There is also strong evidence that acute responses to vigorous physical activity have transient benefits for various domains of cognition such as memory, processing speed, and executive control. These findings are particularly true in children and older adults (14, 15, 18).

There is also evidence for chronic effects of moderate to vigorous physical activity, particularly in individuals over the age of 50 (12,13), and that moderate to vigorous physical activity can improve cognition in individuals who have evidence of impaired cognition particularly related to disorders or diseases such as attention deficit hyperactivity disorder (18), schizophrenia (19), multiple sclerosis (20), Parkinson's disease (21), and stroke (22).

Cognitive function is important for multiple facets of life including academic attainment, job performance, and QoL. There is moderate evidence that greater amounts of physical activity improve these various domains of cognition. The most dramatic improvements in cognitive function with regard to physical activity have been shown to involve executive function (16). The positive effects of physical activity on cognition have been observed in studies involving multiple stages of the lifespan and are particularly present in young children and older adults (23).

11.3   PHYSICAL ACTIVITY AND IMPAIRED
COGNITIVE FUNCTION

A healthy brain is essential for multiple aspects of living a longer and fuller life (12). Aspects of cognitive function such as the ability to plan actions and maintain emotional connections are critically important for an individual's ability to maximize overall QoL and independence (17). Poor brain health may ultimately become manifested as cognitive impairment or dementia and may be associated with underlying disorders including Alzheimer's disease (AD), stroke, other causes of vascular cognitive impairments, brain trauma, and neurodegenerative disorders.

It has been estimated that the United States has the second largest number of people living with dementia (3.9 million people) only exceeded by the largest number of people living with dementia in China (5.4 million people) (24). Worldwide, over 7 million of new cases of dementia are diagnosed annually. By 2050, the prevalence of dementia is expected to increase by over 100% in high-income countries and over 250% in low-income countries. It is estimated that over 10% of adults greater than 60 years of age have memory loss and 35% of those report functional difficulties (25). Over 5 million people in the United States over the age of 65 are estimated to have AD and this is predicted to rise to 13.2 million individuals by 2050 (26).

According to the PAGA 2018 Scientific Report, strong evidence demonstrates that greater amounts of physical activity are associated with reduced risk of cognitive decline and risk of dementia, including AD (1). Furthermore, some evidence indicates that physical activity can improve cognition in individuals who are already suffering from dementia, including AD.

Moderate evidence exists to indicate that increased PA improves cognitive function in individuals with other diseases or disorders impairing cognitive function including ADHD, schizophrenia, multiple sclerosis (MS), Parkinson's disease, and stroke (1).

11.4 PHYSICAL ACTIVITY AND BIOMARKERS OF BRAIN HEALTH

A variety of biomarkers of brain health have been reported to improve with physical activity including neurotropic factors (27), task-evoked brain activity, volume, and connectivity (28–30). Most of these data come from work in children and adults over the age of 60. For example, in the Framingham Study, physical activity was associated with increased total brain volumes in individuals age 60 or older (mean age 70 ± 7 years) (31). In this study, low physical activity (lowest quintile of PA) increased the risk of incident dementia compared to those in higher quintiles by approximately 50%. This suggests that low physical activity is associated with higher risk of dementia in older individuals and that a reduced risk of dementia and higher brain volumes appear to be additional health benefits for maintaining physical activity in old age.

A variety of techniques have been used to look at biomarkers for brain health and cognition. These include gray matter morphology (volume, density, and thickness), white matter integrity, and cortical electrophysiology. Magnetic resonance spectroscopy and positron emission tomography (PET) have also been utilized. This growing body of information suggests that physical activity is associated with 10–70% of improvement in brain outcomes (28, 30).

11.5 PHYSICAL ACTIVITY AND QUALITY OF LIFE

The concept of QoL relates to the way the individuals perceive and react to either their health status or nonmedical aspects of their lives (32). This topic is typically divided into health-related QoL and non-health-related QoL (33). Evidence for the relationship between physical activity and perceived positive QoL is strong. This is particularly true in older adults (over the age of 50 and primarily over the age of 65) and is more strongly related to health-related QoL. The evidence is also strong and also showing that in individuals between the ages of 18 and 65 regular physical activity improves health-related QoL compared to no treatment controls.

The instrument that is typically used to measure QoL is the Short Form Health Survey (SF-36) although other questionnaires have also been utilized. These findings are particularly important given the large number of individuals who report stress in their lives due to a variety of factors such as work, money, and the future of our country. This stress can interfere with daily living and many other aspects of health and could be mitigated by a higher sense of QoL that has been demonstrated to be related to regular physical activity. Thus, physical activity is very important for enabling individuals to lead productive and happy lives with improved QoL.

11.6   PHYSICAL ACTIVITY AND AFFECT

Affect is defined as the subjective experience of feeling states including pleasure/displeasure and arousal (34). According to the PAGA 2018 Scientific Report there is strong evidence that as exercise intensity increases, particularly above the ventilatory threshold, negative affect increases. It should be noted that physical activity is highly effective in reducing acute ("state") anxiety and longer participation in regular physical activity can also reduce "trait" anxiety in both middle-aged and older adults. There is also strong evidence that physical activity can reduce symptoms of depression.

11.7   PHYSICAL ACTIVITY AND ANXIETY

Anxiety may be defined as a "noticeable psychophysical emotional state most often characterized by feelings of apprehension, fear or expectations of fear, worry, nervousness, and physical sensations arising from activation of the autonomic nervous system" (35). The annual prevalence of any anxiety disorder is estimated at 18.1% in the United States with females being 60% more likely than males to experience it.

Anxiety, in general, is a normal and to some degree essential human emotion. For example, it may secure survival by activating fight or flight reactions and signals looming danger thereby protecting individuals from harm. Anxiety is considered pathological when it emerges in situations that are not objectively dangerous or if it is excessively strong or if anticipatory anxiety significantly constrains the life of the affected.

As levels of stress in the modern world have continued to increase, symptoms of anxiety may be elevated even in those without clinical manifestations of anxiety (35).

The positive effects of physical activity on anxiety and anxiety disorders have been frequently studied (34–40). In cross sectional studies, self-reported levels of physical activity have been generally found to result in decreased emotional stress and fewer symptoms of anxiety (37). Regular physical activity has been shown to lower anxiety in healthy individuals (38). Both acute bouts of exercise and chronic levels of physical activity have been shown to reduce "state" anxiety whereas chronic bouts of physical activity have been shown to lower "trait" anxiety (39, 40). Small to moderate amounts of decreased anxiety have also been found in response to resistance strength training (41).

There is also some evidence that regular physical activity may reduce the likelihood of panic disorder and also post-traumatic stress disorder. There is some evidence to suggest that regular physical activity is associated with improved coping skills and increased self-efficacy that often go hand in hand with improving anxiety disorders.

Some evidence also exists suggesting that physical activity deflects negative thoughts. When physical activity is carried out in a group, social interaction may also contribute to relieving anxiety. Some evidence suggests that regular physical activity reduces anxiety by increasing endorphins (41). While this in the past has been largely speculative, recent evidence from PET has shown that decreased levels of anxiety correlated with opioid binding in several brain areas, although these findings must be considered preliminary (41).

11.8   PHYSICAL ACTIVITY AND DEPRESSION

Major depressive disorders (MDD) annually affect approximately 10% of the population in the United States, with a lifetime prevalence in 10% of men and 15% of women (35). The annual economic burden of depressive disorders is estimated at $210 billion. Even in individuals who do not meet diagnostic criteria for MDD, symptoms of depression can have a negative influence on health. Elevated depressive symptoms are associated with increased risk of MDD, functional impairment, high rates of disability, and increased social dysfunction.

Physical activity has been shown to lower the risk of depressive disorders in a number of studies. These include cross-sectional studies and randomized controlled trials (42). There is evidence that there is an inverse relationship between symptoms of depression and physical activity although the complex and multifaceted nature of this relationship mandates that these relationships be treated with caution.

Randomized controlled trials have also shown that both aerobic exercise and resistance strength training can lower the risk of depression. In addition, multiple studies demonstrate that both of these reduce symptoms of depression. Increasing levels of physical activity have been associated with reduced risk of developing depression. There appears to be a dose–response relationship, with more activity associated with larger effects of reducing depression. For example, engaging in more than 30 minutes per day of physical activity reduces the odds of experiencing depression by 48% (43).

With regard to treatment, most studies have explored 12 weeks of physical activity and their effect on depression (44–51). Meta-analyses and systematic reviews of these studies have shown consistent and moderate to large effects of physical activity and depressive symptoms across the adult lifespan. When physical activity is compared with either cognitive behavioral therapies or antidepressant pharmaceutical treatment, studies have shown no differences. This indicates that physical activity is as effective in treating depression as other common approaches to treatment (52). A number of studies have also shown that physical activity reduces depressive symptoms in youth (53).

11.9   PHYSICAL ACTIVITY AND SLEEP

The PAGA 2018 Scientific Report cites strong evidence that both acute and regular bouts of physical activity improve sleep outcomes in adults (1). In addition, moderate evidence was found that physical activity improves sleep outcome across age and sex with the exception that sleep onset latency declines with age even in the presence of increased physical activity.

Sleep is an important determinant of health and well-being across the lifespan (54, 55). Sleep plays an essential role in biological function and is important for neuro development, learning, memory, emotional regulation, and cardiovascular and metabolic health.

A wide variety of studies have looked at various aspects of sleep including sleep latency (the length of time between going to bed and falling asleep), total sleep time, sleep efficiency, sleep quality, day time sleepiness, insomnia, and obstructive sleep apnea (OSA) (54–56). Three meta-analyses and three systematic reviews have all reported beneficial effects of greater amounts of physical activity on one or more aspects of sleep. These studies have consistently shown small to moderate-sized benefits for both regular physical activity and acute bouts of physical activity on a variety of sleep outcomes including total sleep time, sleep efficiency, sleep onset latency, sleep quality, and rapid eye movement sleep (57–62). It should be noted that the time of day in which an acute bout of moderate to vigorous physical activity is performed does not appear to be related to most aspects of sleep.

In adults, physical activity has been shown to improve various sleep outcomes across young, middle aged, and older men and women. There is moderate evidence to suggest that physical activity reduces episodes of OSA, and various aspects of sleep apnea including reduced daytime sleepiness and improved sleep efficiency (63, 64). Apnea hypopnea index, which is the most widely used metric for grading severity of sleep apnea and is the mean number of apneic plus hypopneic events per hour, is also decreased by physical activity (65).

Moderate evidence also indicates a benefit of physical activity on various parameters related to insomnia including improved sleep quality, decreased sleep onset latency, and total awake time after sleep onset (62, 66).

Improvements in sleep carry significant public health impacts. Approximately 10% of adults suffer from clinically diagnosed insomnia (67) and 26% of adults between the ages of 30 and 70 suffer from OSA (68). The prevalence of OSA appears to be rising because a major risk factor for this condition is obesity (69). In addition to these specific disorders, 25% of the population reports getting insufficient sleep on at least 15 out of every 30 days (70) and 25–48% of the population report a sleep problem of some kind.

Sleep problems are also associated with multiple health issues including increased risk of accidents, cardiovascular risk factors, heart disease, obesity, stroke, and all-cause mortality (65). The National Highway Traffic Safety Administration estimates that 2.5% of all fatal vehicle accidents and 2% of nonfatal crashes involve drowsiness while driving (55). Others have suggested that the estimate may be as high as 15–33% (71). It has been estimated that the United States suffers economic losses of up to $411 billion per year as a result of insufficient sleep (31). OSA has strong associations with hypertension, heart failure, obesity, type 2 diabetes, myocardial infarction, stroke, and traffic and industrial accidents.

11.10   PHYSICAL ACTIVITY AND COGNITIVE RESERVE

The robust evidence of multiple benefits of physical activity on the brain throughout the lifespan has caused some investigators to postulate the concept of "cognitive reserve" (72). These investigators maintain that the primary effect of physical activity and exercise on the human brain is to build cognitive reserve (73). Cognitive reserve is hypothesized as the capacity of the mature adult brain to sustain function and resist the effects of disease or injury sufficient to cause a decline in cognition or clinical dementia (74). It is suggested that individuals who experience these declines have less cognitive reserve and that physical activity helps build and maintain this cognitive reserve.

Cognitive reserve is further classified as (1) active reserve and (2) passive reserve. The former refers to the efficiency and adaptability of neural circuits to respond to cognitive challenges as exemplified by compensation and use of other parts of the brain (72). The concept of passive reserve refers to structural anatomic properties such as brain tissue density, white matter integrity, and vascularity. The theory of cognitive reserve is based on a variety of investigations of neurobiology that have explored neurologic factors that are likely to contribute to cognitive reserve. These factors include the correlation of various neurotransmitters, the increase in various neurotrophic factors, e.g. brain-derived neurotrophic factor (75), increase in synaptogenesis (76) (generation of new brain synapses), and neurogenesis (77) (the growth or new neurons in the brain), all of which appear to be related to increased physical activity in humans.

In addition, cerebral blood flow normally decreases with age and dementia. Physical activity has been shown to improve both blood volume and vasculature in the brain (78, 79). This process is called angiogenesis, which is the development of new blood vessels through sprouting of existing vessels and epithelial cells. All of these processes are components of cognitive reserve that are positively affected by physical activity and could help delay the onset of deterioration of cognitive function.

11.11 DEFINING OPTIMAL BRAIN HEALTH

The role of cognitive function and other aspects of brain health is so important that the AHA and the ASA have joined forces to issue a Presidential Advisory defining "optimal" brain health in adults (17). As noted in the AHA/ASA Presidential Advisory, the role of cardiovascular risks have shown them to be closely associated with brain health and to prevent dementia in later life (80, 81). A healthy brain is essential for living a longer and fuller life. Sustaining brain health over the course of a lifetime is important to allow one to maximize one's overall QoL, functional ability, and independence (80, 81). Thus, the impact of maximizing and maintaining brain health has enormous personal and public health implications.

As noted in the joint AHA/ASA Presidential Advisory, most definitions of brain health emphasize absence of overt or vascular or neurodegenerative injuries such as from stroke or AD. Optimum brain health, however, extends this concept to include optimal capacity to function and adapt to the environment. This includes cognition as well as lowering the risk of many other insults to the brain such as stroke (17).

The recommendations from the Presidential Advisory from the AHA/ASA emphasized physical activity as one of the seven metrics to contribute to optimal brain health. This is the same framework that was initially defined by the AHA as "life's simple seven" (82). These include nonsmoking, healthy diet, and weight management (BMI < 25 kg/m^2), and it also placed a strong emphasis on physical activity.

The AHA/ASA Presidential Advisory document also emphasizes that physical activity plays an important role in minimizing other risk factors for heart disease and stroke including high blood pressure. As noted in the Advisory, physically active individuals have a 35% lower risk of cognitive decline compared to those who are physically inactive (83).

It is encouraging to see that both the AHA and the ASA have produced a joint statement indicating that many of the simple activities that can be accomplished in daily life such as physical activity play an important role not only in heart health but also in optimizing brain health.

The role of physical activity in maintaining brain health has important public health implications across many domains. In the area of cognition, multiple studies have shown that physical activity influences cognitive function throughout the lifespan. Maintaining cognitive function is particularly important in older adults. It is estimated that by the year 2050 the population of adults over 65 years in the United States will reach 83.7 million individuals, which is double the 2012 level of 43.1 million (see Chapter 8). Physical activity may be an effective approach to improve cognitive function in this population.

With regard to cognitive decline and AD, the Alzheimer's Disease Foundation has estimated an annual direct cost of AD in the United States is approximately $259 billion (84). It has been estimated that in the last five years of life, the cost of dementia per person was $287,000. It is estimated that costs associated with AD and other dementias may increase to about $785 billion by the year 2050. Physical activity may be a highly effective approach to lowering the risk of developing AD as well as improving function and mitigating costs associated by AD and other cognitive impairments. It has been estimated that approximately 21% of AD cases in the United States are attributed to physical inactivity. A 25% decrease in inactivity could potentially prevent 230,000 cases of AD (84).

With regard to QoL, reductions and low levels of QoL have been linked to mortality risk in older adults and also greater use of health-care services. Moreover, Americans report increasing levels of stress in their lives from a variety of sources. Stress can significantly impair daily function and may be mitigated by a higher sense of QoL. Increased physical activity can help improve QoL and help reduce levels of stress.

With regard to affect, depression, and anxiety, increased levels of physical activity have been demonstrated to improve overall affect and lower the risk of both anxiety and depression throughout the lifespan (40, 42). Both depression and anxiety are very common in the adult population in the United States. Increased physical activity has been shown to be as effective or more effective than pharmaceutical therapy for both of these conditions (51).

11.12 CONCLUSIONS

Physical activity plays a critically important role in multiple aspects of brain health. This includes preservation of cognitive function, as well as decrease in the likelihood of dementias of all kinds including AD. Moreover, physical activity improves QoL and various aspects of affect and mood, and decreases the likelihood of anxiety and depression. Furthermore, physical activity is critically important to multiple aspects of sleep. For all of these reasons, physical activity is one of the most important aspects of improving brain health. Unfortunately, this aspect of physical activity is poorly understood by the public at large. It is hoped that in the future there will be a recognition of the profoundly important aspects of brain health related to physical activity.

CLINICAL APPLICATIONS

- Physicians should emphasize to all patients the important role of physical activity in multiple aspects of brain health.
- Physicians should inquire about physical activity in all patients regardless of age or background.
- Physical activity prescription is important for individuals of all ages and background but particularly important to various aspects of brain health including maintenance of appropriate cognition and decreasing the likelihood of cognitive decline, AD, and other forms of dementia.

REFERENCES

1. 2018 Physical Activity Guidelines Advisory Committee Scientific Report for Americans on Brain Health. Part F Chapter 3 on Brain Health. Washington, DC. 2018.
2. Etnier JL, Nowell PM, Landers DM, Sibley BA. A meta-regression to examine the relationship between aerobic fitness and cognitive performance. Brain Res Rev. 2006;52(1):119–130.
3. Smith PJ, Blumenthal JA, Hoffman BM, et al. Aerobic exercise and neurocognitive performance: a meta-analytic review of randomized controlled trials. Psychosom Med. 2010;72(3):239–252. doi:10.1097/PSY.0b013e3181d14633.
4. Colcombe S, Kramer AF. Fitness effects on the cognitive function of older adults: a meta-analytic study. Psychol Sci. 2003;14(2):125–130.
5. Kelly ME, Loughrey D, Lawlor BA, et al. The impact of exercise on the cognitive functioning of healthy older adults: a systematic review and meta-analysis. Ageing Res Rev. 2014;16:12–31. doi:10.1016/j.arr.2014.05.002.
6. Bustamante EE, Williams CF, Davis CL. Physical activity interventions for neurocognitive and academic performance in overweight and obese youth: a systematic review. Pediatr Clin North Am. 2016;63(3):459–480. doi:10.1016/j.pcl.2016.02.004.
7. Carson V, Hunter S, Kuzik N, et al. Systematic review of physical activity and cognitive development in early childhood. J Sci Med Sport. 2016;19(7):573–578. doi:10.1016/j.jsams.2015.07.011.
8. Donnelly JE, Hillman CH, Castelli D, et al. Physical activity, fitness, cognitive function, and academic achievement in children: a systematic review. Med Sci Sports Exerc. 2016;48(6):1197–1222. doi:10.1249/MSS.000000000000090.
9. Esteban-Cornejo I, Tejero-Gonzalez CM, Sallis JF, Veiga OL. Physical activity and cognition in adolescents: a systematic review. J Sci Med Sport. 2015;18(5):534–539.
10. Tan BWZ, Pooley JA, Speelman CP. A meta-analytic review of the efficacy of physical exercise interventions on cognition in individuals with autism spectrum disorder and ADHD. J Autism Dev Disord. 2016;46(9):3126–3143. doi:10.1007/s10803-016-2854-x.
11. Beckett M, Ardern C, Rotondi M. A meta-analysis of prospective studies on the role of physical activity and the prevention of Alzheimer's disease in older adults. BMC Geriatr. 2015;15:9. doi:10.1186/s12877-015-0007-2.

12. Sofi F, Valecchi D, Bacci D, et al. Physical activity and risk of cognitive decline: a meta-analysis of prospective studies. J Intern Med. 2011;269(1):107–117. doi:10.1111/j.1365-2796.2010.02281.x.

13. Zheng G, Xia R, Zhou W, Tao J, Chen L. Aerobic exercise ameliorates cognitive function in older adults with mild cognitive impairment: a systematic review and meta-analysis of randomised controlled trials. Br J Sports Med. 2016a;50:1443–1450.

14. Chang YK, Labban JD, Gapin JI, Etnier JL. The effects of acute exercise on cognitive performance: a meta-analysis. Brain Res. 2012;1453:87–101. doi:10.1016/j.brainres.2012.02.068.

15. Lambourne K, Tomporowski P. The effect of exercise-induced arousal on cognitive task performance: a meta-regression analysis. Brain Res. 2010;1341:12–24. doi:10.1016/j.brainres.2010.03.091.

16. Ludyga S, Gerber M, Brand S, Holsboer-Trachsler E, Pühse U. Acute effects of moderate aerobic exercise on specific aspects of executive function in different age and fitness groups: a meta-analysis. Psychophysiology. 2016;53(11):1611–1626. doi:10.1111/psyp.12736.

17. Gorelick PB, Furie KL, Iadecola C, et al. Defining optimal brain health in adults: a presidential advisory from the American Heart Association/American Stroke Association. Stroke. 2017;48:e284–e303.

18. Janssen M, Toussaint HM, van Mechelen W, Verhagen EA. Effects of acute bouts of physical activity on children's attention: a systematic review of the literature. Springerplus. 2014;3:410. doi:10.1186/2193-1801-3-410.

19. Firth J, Stubbs B, Rosenbaum S, et al. Aerobic exercise improves cognitive functioning in people with schizophrenia: a systematic review and meta-analysis. Schizophr Bull. 2017;43(3):546–556. doi:10.1093/schbul/sbw115.

20. Morrison JD, Mayer L. Physical activity and cognitive function in adults with multiple sclerosis: an integrative review. Disabil Rehabil. 2016:1–12.

21. Murray DK, Sacheli MA, Eng JJ, Stoessl AJ. The effects of exercise on cognition in Parkinson's disease: a systematic review. Transl Neurodegener. 2014;3(1):5. doi:10.1186/2047-9158-3-5. 10.1186/2047-9158-3-5.

22. Zheng G, Zhou W, Xia R, et al. Aerobic exercises for cognition rehabilitation following stroke: a systematic review. J Stroke Cerebrovasc Dis. 2016b;25(11):2780–2789. doi:10.1016/j.jstrokecerebrovasdis.2016.07.035.

23. MacPherson H, Teo W, Schneider L, Smith A. A life-long approach to physical activity for brain health. Front Aging Neurosci. 2017;(9):1–12.

24. World Health Organization and Alzheimer's Disease International Dementia: a public health priority. Paper presented at World Health Organization; April 11, 2012; Geneva, Switzerland.

25. Centers for Disease Control and Prevention (CDC). Self-reported increased confusion or memory loss and associated functional difficulties among adults aged ≥ 60 years - 21 States, 2011. MMWR Morb Mortal Wkly Rep. 2013;62:347–350.

26. Alzheimer's Association. 2013 Alzheimer's disease facts and figures. Alzheimer's Dementia: J Alzheimer's Assoc. 2013;9:208–245.

27. Fillit HM, Butler RN, O'Connell AW, et al. Achieving and maintaining cognitive vitality with aging. Mayo Clin Proc. 2002;77:681–696.

28. Li MY, Huang MM, Li SZ, et al. The effects of aerobic exercise on the structure and function of DMN-related brain regions: a systematic review. Int J Neurosci. 2016;127(7):634–649.

29. Halloway S, Wilbur J, Schoeny ME, Arfanakis K. Effects of endurance-focused physical activity interventions on brain health: a systematic review. Biol Res Nurs. 2016:19(1):53–64.

30. Sexton CE, Betts JF, Demnitz N, et al. A systematic review of MRI studies examining the relationship between physical fitness and activity and the white matter of the ageing brain. Neuroimage. 2016;131:81–90. doi:10.1016/j.neuroimage.2015.09.071.

31. Tan Z, Spartano N, Beiser A, et al. Physical activity, brain volume, and dementia risk: the Framingham Study. J Gerontol A Biol Sci Med Sci. 2017;72:789–795. doi: 710.1093/gerona/glw1130.

32. Gill T, Feinstein A. A critical appraisal of the quality of quality of life measurements. JAMA. 1994;272(8):619–626.

33. Ware JE Jr, Sherbourne CD. The MOS 36-item short-form health survey (SF-36). Conceptual framework and item selection. Med Care. 1992;30(6):473–483.

34. Russell JA, Barrett LF. Core affect, prototypical emotional episodes, and other things called emotion: dissecting the elephant. J Pers Soc Psychol. 1999;76(5):805–819. doi:10.1037/0022-3514.76.5.805.

35. American Psychiatric Association. Diagnostic and Statistical Manual of Mental Disorders (4th edition, text rev.). American Psychiatric Publishing (Arlington, VA), 2000.

36. Ensari I, Greenlee T, Moti R, et al. Meta-analysis of acute exercise effects on state anxiety: an update of randomized controlled trials over the past 25 years. Depress Anxiety. 2015;32(8): 634–634. doi:10.1002/da.22370.

37. Bartley CA, Hay M, Bloch MH. Meta-analysis: aerobic exercise for the treatment of anxiety disorders. Prog Neuropsychopharmacol Biol Psychiatry. 2013;45(2):34–39. doi:10.1016/j.pnpbp.2013.04.016

38. Mochcovitch MD, Deslandes AC, et al. The effects of regular physical activity on anxiety symptoms in healthy older adults: a systematic review. Rev Bras Psiquiatr. 2016;38(3):255–261.

39. Jayakody K, Gunadasa S, Hosker C. Exercise for anxiety disorders: systematic review. Br J Sports Med. 2014;48(3):187–196. doi:10.1136/bjsports-2012-091287.

40. Stonerock GL, Hoffman BM, Smith PJ, Blumenthal JA. Exercise as treatment for anxiety: systematic review and analysis. Ann Behav Med. 2015;49(4):542–556. doi:10.1007/s12160-014-9685-9.

41. Gordon BR, McDowell CP, Lyons M, et al. The effects of resistance exercise training on anxiety: a meta-analysis and meta-regression analysis of randomized controlled trials. Sports Med. 2017;47:2521–2532.

42. Mammen G, Faulkner G Physical activity and the prevention of depression: a systematic review of prospective studies. Am J Prev Med. 2013;45(5):649–657. doi:10.1016/j.amepre.2013.08.001.

43. Zhai L, Zhang Y, Zhang D. Sedentary behaviour and the risk of depression: a meta-analysis. Br J Sports Med. 2015;49(11):705–709. doi:10.1136/bjsports-2014-093613.

44. Robertson R, Robertson A, Jepson R, Maxwell M. Walking for depression or depressive symptoms: a systematic review and meta-analysis. Ment Health Phys Act. 2012;5(1):66–75.

45. de Souza Moura AM, Lamego MK, Paes F, et al. Effects of aerobic exercise on anxiety disorders: a systematic review. CNS Neurol Disord Drug Targets. 2015;14(9):1184–1193. doi:10.2174/1871527315666151111121259.

46. Nystrom MB, Neely G, Hassmen P, Carlbring P. Treating major depression with physical activity: a systematic overview with recommendations. Cogn Behav Ther. 2015;44(4):341–352.

47. Rebar AL, Stanton R, Geard D, et al. A meta-meta-analysis of the effect of physical activity on depression and anxiety in non-clinical adult populations. Health Psychol Rev. 2015;9(3):366–378. doi:10.1080/17437199.2015.1022901.

48. Yan S, Jin Y, Oh Y, Choi Y. Effect of exercise on depression in university students: a meta-analysis of randomized controlled trials. J Sports Med Phys Fitness. 2016;56(6):811–816.

49. Josefsson T, Lindwall M, Archer T. Physical exercise intervention in depressive disorders: metaanalysis and systematic review. Scand J Med Sci Sports. 2014;24(2):259–272. doi:10.1111/sms.12050.

50. Schuch FB, Vancampfort D, Richards J et al. Exercise as a treatment for depression: a meta-analysis adjusting for publication bias. J Psychiatr Res. 2016b;77:42–51. doi:10.1016/j.jpsychires.2016.02.023.

51. Farah WH, Alsawas, M, Mainou M, et al. Non-pharmacological treatment of depression: a systematic review and evidence map. Evid Based Med. 2016;21(6):214–221.

52. Lindheimer JB, O'Connor PJ, Dishman RK. Quantifying the placebo effect in psychological outcomes of exercise training: a meta-analysis of randomized trials. Sports Med. 2015;45(5):693–711. doi:10.1007/s40279-015-0303-1.

53. Brown H, Pearson N, Braithwaite R, et al. Physical activity interventions and depression in children and adolescents: a systematic review and meta-analysis. Sports Med. 2013;43:195–206. doi:10.1007/s40279-012-0015-8.

54. Office of Disease Prevention and Health Promotion. Sleep Health. Office of Disease Prevention and Health Promotion (Washington, DC), 2017. https://www.healthypeople.gov/2020/topicsobjectives/topic/sleep-health.

55. Mukherjee S, Patel SR, Kales SN, et al. An official American thoracic society statement: the importance of healthy sleep. Recommendations and future priorities. Am J Respir Crit Care Med. 2015;191(12):1450–1458. doi:10.1164/rccm.201504-0767ST.

56. Berry RB, Brooks R, Gamaldo CE, et al. The AASM Manual for the Scoring of Sleep and Associated Events: Rules, Terminology and Technical Specifications, Version 2.4. American Academy of Sleep Medicine (Darien, IL), 2017.

57. Kredlow MA, Capozzoli MC, et al. The effects of physical activity on sleep: a meta-analytic review. J Behav Med. 2015;38(3):427–449. doi:10.1007/s10865-015-9617-6.

58. Lang C, Kalak N, Brand S, et al. The relationship between physical activity and sleep from mid adolescence to early adulthood. A systematic review of methodological approaches and meta-analysis. Sleep Med Rev. 2016;28:32–45. doi:10.1016/j.smrv.2015.07.004.

59. Rubio-Arias JÁ, Marín-Cascales E, Ramos-Campo DJ, et al. Effect of exercise on sleep quality and insomnia in middle-aged women: a systematic review and meta-analysis of randomized controlled trials. Maturitas. 2017;100:49–56. doi:10.1016/j.maturitas.2017.04.003.

60. Yang PY, Ho KH, Chen HC, Chien MY. Exercise training improves sleep quality in middle-aged and older adults with sleep problems: a systematic review. J Physiother. 2012;58(3):157–163. doi:10.1016/S1836-9553(12)70106-6.

61. Dolezal BA, Neufeld EV, Boland DM, et al. Interrelationship between sleep and exercise: a systematic review. Adv Prev Med. 2017;2017:1364387. doi:10.1155/2017/1364387.

62. Passos GS, Poyares DL, Santana MG, et al. Is exercise an alternative treatment for chronic insomnia. Clinics (Sao Paulo). 2012;67(6):653–660.

63. Iftikhar IH, Bittencourt L, Youngstedt SD, et al. Comparative efficacy of CPAP, MADs, exercise training, and dietary weight loss for sleep apnea: a network meta-analysis. Sleep Med. 2017;30:7–14. doi:10.1016/j.sleep.2016.06.001.

64. Iftikhar IH, Kline CE, Youngstedt SD. Effects of exercise training on sleep apnea: a meta-analysis. Lung. 2014;192(1):175–184. 10.1007/s00408-013-9511-3.

65. Greenberg DL. Obstructive sleep apnea. In Kryger MH, Roth T, Dement WC. Principles and Practice of Sleep Medicine (5th edition). Elsevier Saunders (St. Louis), 2017.

66. Smagula SF, Stone KL, Fabio A, Cauley JA. Risk factors for sleep disturbances in older adults: evidence from prospective studies. Sleep Med Rev. 2016;25:21–30. doi:10.1016/j.smrv.2015.01.003.

67. Institute of Medicine, Committee on Sleep Medicine and Research. Sleep Disorders and Sleep Deprivation: An Unmet Public Health Problem. National Academies Press (Washington, DC), 2006.

68. Peppard PE, Young T, Barnet JH, et al. Increased prevalence of sleep-disordered breathing in adults. Am J Epidemiol. 2013;177(9):1006–1014.
69. American Academy of Sleep Medicine. Rising Prevalence of Sleep Apnea in U.S. Threatens Public Health. American Academy of Sleep Medicine (Washington, DC), 2014. https://aasm.org/risingprevalence-of-sleep-apnea-in-u-s-threatens-public-health/.
70. Centers for Disease Control and Prevention, Epidemiology Program Office. Perceived insufficient rest or sleep among adults: United States, 2008. MMWR. 2009;58(42):1175–1179.
71. Hafner M, Stepanek M, Taylor J, et al. Why Sleep Matters—The Economic Costs of Insufficient Sleep: A Cross-Country Comparative Analysis. Rand Corp (Cambridge, UK), 2016.
72. Kayes M, Hatfield B. Influence of physical activity on brain aging and cognition: The role of cognitive reserve, thresholds for decline, genetic influence, and the investment hypothesis. In Rippe JM: Lifestyle Medicine (3rd edition). CRC Press (Boca Raton, FL), 2019.
73. Scarmeas N, Stern Y. Cognitive reserve and lifestyle. J Clin Exp Neuropsychol. 2003;25:625–633.
74. Rovio S, Kareholt I, Helkala E, et al. Leisure-time physical activity at midlife and the risk of dementia and Alzheimer's disease. Lancet Neurol. 2005;4: 705–711.
75. Neeper SA, Gomez-Pinilla F, Choi J, Cotman C. Exercise and brain neurotrophins Nature. 1995;373:109.
76. Vaynman S, Gomez-Pinilla F. License to run: exercise impacts functional plasticity in the intact and injured central nervous system by using neurotrophins. Neurorehabil Neural Repair. 2005;19: 283–295.
77. van Praag H, Christie BR, Sejnowski TJ, Gage FH. Running enhances neurogenesis, learning, and long-term potentiation in mice. Proc Natl Acad Sci. 1999;96: 13427–13431.
78. van de Borght K, Kobor-Nyakaa DE, Klauke K, et al. Physical exercise leads to rapid adaptations in hippocampal vasculature: temporal dynamics and relationship to cell proliferation and neurogenesis. Hippocamp. 2009;19: 928–936,.
79. Palmer TD, Willhoite AR, Gage FH. Vascular niche for adult hippocampal neurogenesis. J Comp Neurol. 2000;425:479–494.
80. Fiocco AJ, Yaffe K. Defining successful aging: the importance of including cognitive function over time Arch. Neurol. 2010;67:876–880.
81. Centers for Disease Control and Prevention, Healthy Aging. What is a healthy brain?. New research explores perceptions of cognitive health among diverse older adults. https://www.cdc.gov/aging/pdf/perceptions_of_cog_hlth_factsheet.pdf   [Accessed January 27, 2020].
82. American Heart Association. Life's Simple 7. https://www.heart.org/en/healthy-living/healthy-lifestyle/my-life-check–lifes-simple-7. [Accessed February 3, 2020].
83. Blondell SJ, Hammersley-Mather R, Veerman JL. Does physical activity prevent cognitive decline and dementia? A systematic review and meta-analysis of longitudinal studies. BMC Public Health. 2014; 14:510.
84. Hurd MD, Martorell P, Delavande A, et al. Monetary costs of dementia in the United States. N Engl J Med. 2013;368:1326–1334.

12 The Role of Physicians in Promoting and Prescribing Increased Physical Activity

KEY POINTS

- Only 20% of the adult population meets the recommended levels of physical activity from the Physical Activity Guidelines for Americans 2018 Scientific Report.
- Only 40% of physicians typically counsel patients in the area of physical activity.
- Physician counseling has been demonstrated to be one of the most powerful methods of encouraging patients to make positive lifestyle decisions.
- Since more than 70% of individuals see their primary care physician at least once a year, this represents a great opportunity to increase the likelihood of patients engaging in physical activity levels.
- Increased physical activity levels among physicians themselves can yield a variety of personal health benefits and also increase the likelihood that they will counsel their patients about physical activity.

12.1 INTRODUCTION

Overwhelming data now exist that regular physical activity yields multiple benefits for both short- and long-term health and quality of life (1). Regular physical activity reduces the risk factors for many chronic diseases such as coronary heart disease (CHD), type 2 diabetes (T2DM), some cancers, metabolic syndrome, and many other conditions (1, 2). In addition, regular physical activity serves as an adjunct in the treatment of many chronic diseases. This fact is recognized and included in the guidelines from virtually every professional organization that deals with chronic metabolic disease (3).

As a cardiologist and lifetime exerciser, I have been both professionally and personally committed to regular physical activity. I am not only familiar with the multiple benefits of regular physical activity that have been documented in literally thousands of studies, but also have seen the benefits of my program of regular physical activity throughout my lifetime. In addition, my research organization, Rippe Lifestyle Institute (RLI), has included regular physical activity as a key component of virtually every study that we have performed over the last 25 years and every patient we have

137

seen in our clinic. Regular physical activity is also a key component that we combine with other lifestyle factors in our various lifestyle medicine publications.

Despite the well-documented benefits of physical activity, sadly the medical community has not been as active as it should have been in the promotion and prescription of regular physical activity. A number of studies have shown that 40% or less of physicians include discussions of regular physical activity in office visits with patients (4). This is a missed opportunity since over 70% of individuals in the United States see their primary care physician at least on an annual basis.

It has been a struggle to get people to engage in meaningful amounts of physical activity. It has been estimated that over 80% of adults in the United States do not meet current physical activity guidelines promulgated by the Physical Activity Guidelines for Americans (PAGA 2018) (Figure 12.1).

These estimates may be even more disheartening when it comes to adolescents. In addition to the known benefits of regular physical activity, there is also increasing evidence that an inactive lifestyle contributes to multiple, long-term adverse health complications. The World Health Organization has ranked physical inactivity as the fourth leading cause of death worldwide (5).

Physician recommendation remains a very powerful motivator to encourage people to make behavioral changes. In fact, a number of studies have shown that physician counseling is the most powerful force for helping people make changes on their habits and practices. Thus, there is a clear mandate for physicians to become involved in recommending increased physical activity to every patient they see (6).

The purpose of this chapter is to provide a general framework and overall guidance to help clinicians increase counseling and recommendations for increased physical activity for every patient.

12.2   THE ROLE OF PHYSICAL ACTIVITY IN LIFESTYLE MEDICINE

While many factors related to daily habits and actions exert powerful impacts on health and quality of life, physical activity is arguably the most important of all these factors. In fact, in the area of cardiovascular medicine an inactive lifestyle is a more powerful predictor of cardiovascular disease (CVD) than any other risk factor including hypertension, dyslipidemia, and obesity (7). The field of lifestyle medicine has grown dramatically over the past two decades. I was pleased to have named this field with the publication of my first academic textbook in this area in 1999 (*Lifestyle Medicine*, Blackwell Science, Inc. (London), 1999) (8). Subsequently, a number of organizations have adopted the framework of lifestyle medicine to describe the importance of lifestyle choices in maintaining good health (9). Though there are multiple components that contribute to positive health, this chapter will focus largely on physical activity.

12.3   PHYSICAL ACTIVITY PROMOTION AND INVOLVEMENT OF PHYSICIANS AND OTHER HEALTH-CARE PROFESSIONALS

The world is in the midst of an epidemic of noncommunicable diseases. In the 1900s, communicable diseases, such as infectious disease, resulted in the top three causes of death in the United States, accounting for 30% of all deaths (10). In

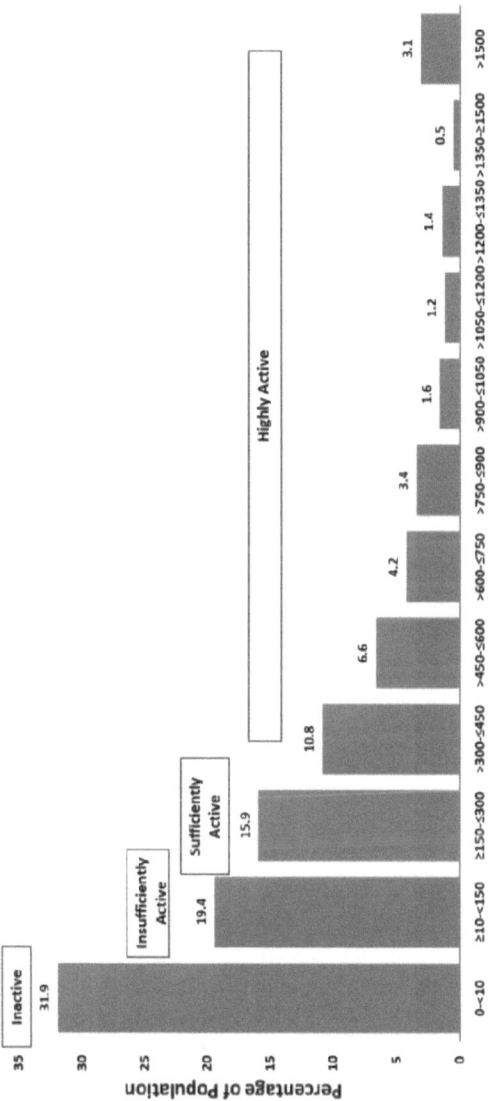

FIGURE 12.1 Distribution of self-reported volume of moderate-to-vigorous physical activity, 150 minutes per week increments, US adults, 2015.

Physical Activity Guidelines Advisory Committee. 2018 Physical Activity Guidelines Advisory Committee. 2018 Physical Activity Committee Scientific Report. Washington, DC US Department of Health and Human Services; 2018. (Adapted from data found in the National Interview Survey, 2015.)

contrast, by 2014, seven out of the top ten causes of death are attributable to chronic, noncommunicable diseases (11). For example, heart disease and cancer represent over 46% of all deaths each year in the United States and also represent the majority of health-care expenditures in the United States (12). In 2010, more than 85% of the $3 trillion spent on health care was spent on chronic diseases (13). It has been suggested that poor lifestyle habits and actions contribute to 75–80% of chronic diseases. Thus, there is no longer any doubt that dealing with lifestyle issues, in general, and physical activity, in particular, represents important target for medical intervention.

12.4   CALLS FOR MORE PHYSICIAN AND OTHER HEALTH-CARE PROFESSIONALS' INVOLVEMENT FOR RECOMMENDING PHYSICAL ACTIVITY

In retrospect, much of the emphasis on lifestyle factors and health may be traced back to the clarion call issued by the then US Surgeon General Julius Richmond in 1979 in his report "Healthy People: The Surgeon General's Report on Health Promotion and Disease Prevention" (14). Increased physical activity was a major theme in this report as well as the strong recommendation that the health-care sector lead in the promotion of this activity.

The Healthy People reports have been subsequently issued and updated in every decade. Though some changes in emphasis have occurred, the importance of physical activity has remained a central focus. Healthy People 2020 lists a number of recommendations concerning the importance of regular physical activity including the recommendation to increase the proportion of physician office visits in both children and adults where recommendations to increase exercise occur (15).

The initial framework for the Healthy People 2030 (16) includes recommendation to improve environments such as sidewalks, bike lanes, trails, and parks that increase the likelihood of physical activity. This framework also targets both schools and childcare settings, as well as work places, as important venues where increased physical activity can be fostered. In all of these settings increased physician involvement is emphasized as an important component of improving levels of physical activity for the population.

A number of specific recommendations related to physical activity were made in the Healthy People 2020 document including encouraging the proportion of adults who engage in aerobic physical activity of at least moderate intensity to 150 (plus) minutes per week and increasing the proportion of adults who performed muscle strengthening activities two or more days per week. Similar objectives were listed for adolescents. In addition, the recommendation was made to increase the proportion of the elementary schools that require daily physical education for all students as well as increasing the number of adolescents who participate in daily school physical education. Many other recommendations were listed in the Healthy People 2020 document for increased physical activity that are consistent with other national guidelines.

12.5   PHYSICAL ACTIVITY RECOMMENDATIONS: THE NATIONAL PERSPECTIVE

The first U.S. National Activity Plan was released in 2010 and subsequently updated in 2016 (17). The health-care sector was identified as one of the nine major areas of focus identified in both of these plans. Included are the recommendations to prioritize efforts in health care to promote physical activity as well as recognizing physical inactivity as both preventable and treatable with both health and cost implications. The National Activity Plans also emphasize the importance of collaborating across sectors and expanding education in the area of physical activity in the training of all health-care professionals.

12.6   THE ROLE OF PROFESSIONAL ORGANIZATIONS IN PROMOTING PHYSICAL ACTIVITY

A number of professional organizations have been become involved in recommending and promoting increased levels of physical activity. Perhaps the most prominent organization in this area is the American College of Sports Medicine (ACSM), which has been the professional home for exercise physiologists and other health-care professionals with a particular interest in exercise for many decades (18). Recently, ACSM has joined forces with the American Medical Association in an initiative titled "Exercise Is Medicine (EIM)" (4). The stated goal of EIM is "for the healthcare community to make physical activity a standard part of the medical paradigm for the prevention and treatment of non-communicable diseases (NCDs) in healthcare systems." This initiative, which was initially launched in the United States, has now spread to more than 40 countries. What started as an initiative to increase awareness about the important health benefits of increased physical activity, the focus has now broadened to include implementation of standard models to help primary care physicians prescribe physical activity as well as linking patients to community resources. The EIM initiative has also provided tools to help guide physicians through the steps to increase physical activity including their "Healthcare Providers Action Guide." This is a free resource that can be downloaded from the EIM website, as well as other resources.

Other professional organizations such as the American College of Lifestyle Medicine (ACLM), American Academy of Geriatrics, American College of Preventive Medicine, the American Academy of Pediatrics, and the American Academy of Orthopedic Surgeons have all issued statements encouraging their members to address physical activity with patients (19).

The American Heart Association (AHA) has also been a leader in emphasizing the importance of lifestyle actions, such as physical activity, in the prevention of CVD. In fact, one of the Councils of the AHA actually changed its name in 2013 from the "Council on Nutrition, Physical Activity and Metabolism" to the "Council on Lifestyle and Cardiometabolic Health" (20). Lifestyle has been emphasized as a key component both in the improvement of lipids and in the control of blood pressure in documents and Scientific Statements issued by the AHA. In 2013, the AHA and the American College of Cardiology issued Guidelines for Lifestyle Management to reduce cardiovascular risk that included a major emphasis on physical activity in lipid management, blood pressure management, and in combination with proper nutrition for weight management (21).

12.7 RATIONALE FOR MORE PHYSICIAN INVOLVEMENT

A number of studies have shown that physicians play a unique role in influencing patient behavior. These studies have demonstrated that physicians are the most trusted source of physical activity information and that patients prefer to receive their initial advice regarding physical activity from their physician as opposed to other health-care providers such as nurses, physical therapists, or dietitians (22–24). In addition, there is evidence that a physician's advice may serve as a catalyst for change by making patients more aware of health information and programs by making the information more relevant (25).

Since over 70% of adults see their primary care physician each year, physicians can play a powerful role in recommending physical activity (26–28). There seems to be some progress in this area, although a distinct minority of physicians still recommend physical activity to their patients. In 2010, only 32% of adults who saw physicians were advised about physical activity, although more recent studies have suggested that up to 40% of patients who see physicians have received recommendations for increased physical activity (29).

12.8 EDUCATIONAL RESOURCES

Multiple educational resources now exist to provide physicians and other health-care workers with evidence-based information concerning various aspects of physical activity. Unfortunately, within the confines of formal medical education physical activity is often underemphasized (30). In fact in 2012, a systematic review of behavior change counseling and curricula in medical schools showed that increased physical activity was the least addressed topic of all health behaviors reviewed following smoking, nutrition, alcohol/drug use (31). In 2014, a systematic review showed that only 11 programs existed that focused on physical activity counseling and these programs were inconsistent with regard to program duration and placement within the curriculum (32). These results suggest that medical students and other physicians who undergo training do not achieve adequate levels of training with respect to prescribing physical activity (33).

Multiple professional organizations and documents are currently available to provide education in the area of physical activity. Perhaps the most comprehensive, evidence-based document for recommendation comes from the (PAGA 2018) (2). This extensive, evidence-based document provides a comprehensive documentation of the benefits of regular physical activity in multiple population groups throughout the lifespan and summarizes the scientific literature with extensive background references.

ACSM also provides abundant tools for practicing physicians and their patients regarding physical activity. The ACLM and also the ACSM provide education in various aspects of lifestyle medicine through their Lifestyle Medicine Education

Collaborative (LMEd) (34). This program, which was created in 2013, has now been accessed by half of all medical schools. The LMEd program also has supplied a collection of peer-reviewed curricula materials through the Med Ed platform that is maintained by the Association of American Medical Colleges.

Finally, CME opportunities exist in the area of physical activity promotion. These will be enumerated at the end of this chapter.

12.9   PHYSICAL ACTIVITY AND FITNESS EVALUATION

The vast majority of individuals who wish to increase the amount of physical activity in their lives may do so without a formal evaluation. This is the position that is also supported by the PAGA 2018 Scientific Report and ACSM (18). Of course, every physician should discuss the importance of physical activity safety and the benefits of physical activity with all patients. There may also be times when particular clinical circumstances would warrant a more formal evaluation. This may be particularly true in individuals with a history of CHD or individuals who have been extremely inactive. In these settings, a variety of potential activity or fitness evaluations are appropriate.

It should also be noted that physical activity and fitness are slightly different terms and have different definitions. ACSM defines physical fitness as "a set of physical attributes that people have or achieve that relate to the ability to perform physical activity" (17). Physical activity is a less formal concept that involves both activities of daily living and low to moderate intensity activities such as walking at three miles an hour or less.

When the clinician feels that an evaluation would be appropriate prior to recommending increased physical activity there are a wide variety of tests available, most of which can be performed either in an office setting or in a cardiology clinic.

These tests include a variety of protocols. Probably the most commonly used protocol is called the Bruce protocol, named after the cardiologist who first developed the protocol. In this protocol, an individual is asked to walk on a treadmill at progressively faster speeds and both the speed and the incline of the treadmill are increased every three minutes. Other protocols include the Balke protocol, where an individual walks on a treadmill at a constant walking speed, while the slope of the treadmill is increased every 1–2 minutes. For men, the treadmill speed for the Balke protocol is specifically set 3.3 miles per hour, after one minute the incline of the treadmill is raised 2%, then 1% each minute thereafter. For women the treadmill speed is typically set at 3.0 miles per hour with a gradient starting at 0% and increased 2.5% every three minutes.

Other protocols may be used in cardiac rehabilitation such as a modified Balke protocol where treadmill speeds are set at a lower speed and inclines are also more gradually increased. Other exercise protocols include a cycle ergometer protocol where workload is increased every two minutes, or a ramp protocol where a constant speed is utilized and the incline of the treadmill progressively increased rather than changing either the speed or grade of protocol in the conventional Balke or Bruce protocols.

All of these tests may be utilized to estimate aerobic fitness. They may be conducted to either a maximum heart rate (maximal texting) or submaximal based on heart rates to achieve submaximal levels. A complete description of protocols utilized for this type of exercise testing is beyond the scope of this chapter, but may be found in a number of publications from the ACSM.

Other types of tests have been utilized to estimate either cardiorespiratory fitness or functional status of patients with cardiovascular or pulmonary disease. These include a six minute walk test, the Cooper twelve minute test, the 1.5 mile test, or the one mile fitness walking test. My research team developed the one mile fitness walking test. The protocols for these tests may be found in a variety of settings and are beyond the scope of this chapter.

Finally, it may be appropriate in some patients to take non-exercise tests to estimate cardiorespiratory fitness. These pencil and paper tests are typically based on utilizing regression equations including age, gender, BMI and, self-reported physical activity patterns, although some other health metrics may also be employed. These equations have been shown to have a reasonably robust correlation with objective fitness measures. A review of these protocols may be found in various ACSM publications (17, 18, 35).

In addition to aerobic fitness, a variety of other fitness measures may be appropriate including muscular strength and endurance and body composition.

In our research laboratory and clinic, we typically utilize both submaximal and maximal aerobic testing, and also a variety of different tests to determine body composition (percentage of body fat and lean muscle). While we are fortunate to have technology including dual-energy X-ray absorptiometry (DEXA), most physicians' offices, as a practical matter, will use body mass index (BMI). This is based on the ratio of weight in kilograms divided by the height and meters.[2] Since the BMI is the simplest and least expensive method of estimating an individual's obesity level, it is widely used in many national studies. The criteria for normal weight, overweight, and obesity in national classifications of these terms utilizes BMI (more detail on this is found in Chapter 10).

12.10   PHYSICAL ACTIVITY AND EXERCISE PRESCRIPTION

The general guidance for physical activity for most healthy, although inactive patients, may be summarized with the phrase of "some is better than none." As illustrated in Chapter 1, there is a steep benefit for lowering all-cause mortality even at very low levels of physical activity. A 20% reduction in all-cause mortality with physical activity may be found at as low as 30 minutes per week, although 75% of the benefit will come for individuals who exercise 150–300 minutes per week (roughly 30–60 minutes on most, if not all, days) (36).

For the safety of patients, it is best to follow recognized training principles that involve slow progression of increases of physical activity. Most people will feel most comfortable in engaging in physical activity on alternate days, although aerobic physical activity may be prescribed at 30 minutes on most, if not all, days. At least a day in between musculoskeletal sessions is optimal.

The intensity level of exercise for most individuals should be "moderate." A reasonable way of assessing this may be to recommend to patients that they should feel that they are exercising enough to slightly sweat, but they should not be exercising harder than would allow them to carry on a normal conversation if the goal is "moderate physical activity." Another way of determining exercise intensity is based on heart rate. There are many different equations available to estimate heart rate. Probably the one that is most widely used is the equation 220 minus age, which predicts maximum heart rate. Then take 50–70% of that, which would constitute moderate intensity physical activity.

A measurement that is used frequently throughout the PAGA 2018 Scientific Report and many ACSM documents (2, 35) is "METs." A "MET" is shorthand for a metabolic equivalent. One MET is the amount of energy expended while sitting at rest. This is the equivalent of about 3.3 milliliters of oxygen per kilogram per minute of body weight. Moderate intensity MET levels are typically 3.0–5.9 METs, whereas vigorous activity is greater than 6 METs. MET level for some common types of physical activity and exercise are listed in Table 12.1 (37).

In addition to aerobic conditioning and musculoskeletal strength training, flexibility training is also recommended by ACSM and it usually involves static activity, where a person holds a stretch for an extended period of time (15 seconds or more). Before and after physical activity, it is also important to warm-up and cooldown. At least five minutes of warm-up and five minutes of cooldown will be helpful in terms of increasing blood flow and body temperature, muscle and connective tissue in warm up, or decreasing these parameters during cool down, thus reducing the chance of injury during vigorous activity. Warm-up and cooldown is less important for moderate intensity physical activity such as walking at 3.5 miles per hour.

TABLE 12.1
Sample Metabolic Equivalent (MET) Levels of Common Physical Activities*

Activity	METs	Activity	METs
Walking, 2 miles per hour	2.8	Aerobic dancing	5.0–9.5
Walking, 3 miles per hour	3.5	Golf, using power cart	3.5
Walking, 4 miles per hour	5.0	Golf, walking, pulling/carrying clubs	4.3–5.3
Running, 6 miles per hour	9.8	Tennis	4.5–8.0
Running, 7.5 miles per hour	11.5	Soccer	7.0–10.0
Running, 9 miles per hour	12.8	Washing and waxing car	2.0
Bicycling, 5.5 miles per hour	3.5	Most housecleaning activities	2.5–3.5
Bicycling, 9.4 miles per hour	5.8	Gardening	2.3–5.8
Bicycling, 15 miles per hour	10.0	Mowing lawn, riding mower	2.5
Swimming, sidestroke	7.0	Mowing lawn, walk, power mower	4.5–5.0
Swimming, crawl, ~50 yards per min	8.3	Mowing lawn, walk, hand mower	6.0
Swimming, crawl, ~75 yards per min	10.0	Shoveling dirt or snow	5.3–7.8

* Adapted from Ainsworth BE, Haskell WL, Hermann SD, et al. The Compendium of Physical Activities Tracking Guide. Healthy Lifestyles Research Center, College of Nursing and Health Innovation, Arizona State University. https://sites.google.com/site/compendiumofphysicalactivities/

Davis PG: Exercise Prescription for Apparently Healthy Individuals and for Special Populations. In Rippe JM: Lifestyle Medicine, 3rd ed. CRC Press (Boca Raton), 2019. (37)

(Used with permission of the editor of Lifestyle Medicine 3rd edition, Dr. James Rippe).

One further aspect of physical activity prescription of great importance is activity adherence. A variety of techniques have been used to increase the likelihood of people adhering to exercise. This is probably best achieved when individuals have tried a variety of different forms of exercises and focused on one that they particularly enjoy the most. Sometimes people find that exercising or engaging in bouts of physical activity with other individuals also increases the likelihood that they will stick with an exercise program.

12.11   PHYSICAL ACTIVITY AND EXERCISE PRESCRIPTION FOR SPECIAL POPULATIONS

In general, the same recommendations of trying to achieve 150 minutes of moderate intensity aerobic physical activity and two weekly sessions of muscular strength training apply to most individuals.

Some modifications may be necessary in some populations and populations with special needs (see Chapters 8 and 9). For example, the PAGA 2018 Scientific Report recommends that children try to accumulate 60 minutes of moderate physical activity on most, if not all, days. Older adults (over the age of 65) can typically try to achieve the 150 minutes of moderate intensity physical activity per week, but may also supplement aerobic physical activities with balance exercises 2–3 days a week to improve balance and decrease the risk of falling.

Physical activity for most women is the same as for men (see Chapter 6). During pregnancy and postpartum, however, there may be some slight modifications, although the typical guideline of 150 minutes of moderate intensity physical activity per week will be appropriate for most individuals. These special populations are handled in various chapters throughout this book with more details concerning physical activity and exercise recommendations for each group.

12.12   GETTING STARTED

For clinicians who wish to get started or who have not previously recommended increased physical activity for their patients, here are a few guidelines that may help starting the process.

First, simply inquiring about current level of physical activity is an excellent start. As already indicated, only 40% of physicians actually inquire about physical activity. Second, utilizing a simple, two-question tool may help initiate this conversation. This part of the initiative incorporated by both the U.S. National Physical Activity Program (19) and the EIM (4) involves utilizing a tool consisting of two questions:

1.) On average, how many days per week do you engage in moderate or strenuous physical activity (like a brisk walk)?
2.) On average, how many minutes do you engage in exercise at this level?

When these two numbers are multiplied with each other, a physician can get an approximation of how close the patient comes to meeting the 150 minutes per week of moderate intensity physical activity recommended by the PAGA 2018, ACSM, AHA, and many other professional organizations.

An additional optional third question recommended by EIM is "How many days a week do you perform muscle strengthening exercises, such as body weight exercise or resistance training?"

Though these questions provide only a basic understanding of the level of physical activity for patients, they have the advantage of being quick and fit quite well into the electronic medical record system. These questions have already been utilized as part of including physical activity vital signs in the system of usual care in a variety of health-care systems.

Once these data are available, the physician can move on to provide a physical activity prescription. As already discussed, this involves the concepts of the frequency, intensity, time and type (FITT), utilizing the following, specific concepts:

- Frequency, how often the activity should be done.
- Intensity, how hard the activity should feel.
- Time, how many minutes the activity should be completed.
- Type, what activities are most appropriate for this patient.

Templates are available through the EIM program to help with exercise prescription that incorporates this framework.

12.13   UTILIZING EXPERTS

Many experts are available to help physicians in the goal of increasing physical activity for patients. A physician may refer to a professional such as an exercise physiologist or to a health club or local YMCA. To assure that a physical activity referral is given to a professional with appropriate credentials, it may be useful to inquire about the ACSM Registered Clinical Exercise Physiologist (RCEP) certification (18). This is the gold standard for individuals prescribing physical activity or exercise programs and identifies people who have a minimum of a master's degree in exercise science and 600 documented hours of experience in a variety of content areas that allow patients to be prescribed regular physical activity. Individuals with ACSM-RCEP must have a current CPR certification and pass a rigorous examination testing their knowledge and skill levels (38).

If a patient is referred to a local health club or YMCA, the patient should inquire about the background and skills of the exercise professionals at each of these locations. A physician may also make those inquiries and refer patients to individuals within these organizations that have the appropriate background level and skill sets.

12.14   BE A ROLE MODEL

Physicians should strive to serve as a role model in the area of physical activity for their patients. A number of studies have shown that there is a strong relationship between a physician's personal health habits and his/her related counseling practices (39). This is true in a variety of areas such as smoking cessation, vaccination, and screening practices, and appears to hold true for physical activity counseling as well.

One review including 24 studies demonstrated an 80% correlation between physicians' personal physical activity habits and their counseling practices (33). Moreover, patient perceptions of the physicians' physical activity behaviors appear to play a role in whether or not the patient engages in physical activity.

Finally, there are emerging data that physicians' physical activity helps reduce the likelihood of physician burnout. Burnout has been described as "a syndrome of emotional exhaustion, loss of meaningful work, feelings of ineffectiveness and a tendency to view people as objects rather than human beings" (40). Unfortunately, over half of US physicians reported experiencing substantial symptoms of burnout. One study of 80 internal medicine residents showed that residents who reported meeting US guidelines for physical activity were significantly less likely to experience burnout than those who failed to achieve recommended levels of physical activity (41, 42).

12.15 RESOURCES

A wide variety of resources are available to assist physicians in gaining knowledge on physical activity and conferring that knowledge to their patients. The following are highly recommended:

- PAGA 2018 Advisory Committee Scientific Report available through https://health.gov/paguidelines/second-edition/report/pdf/PAG_Advisory_Committee_Report.pdf
- ACLM Annual Conference, online CMEs, and residency curriculum available at LifestyleMedicine.org.
- Lifestyle Medicine Education Collaborative Curricula Resources, plus webinars available at LifestyleMedicineEducation.org.
- Multiple ACSM books and other educational resources.

12.16 CONCLUSIONS

Given the low level of physical activity found in the general population in the United States, it is imperative that the medical community, in general, and physicians, in particular, become involved in recommending physical activity to all patients. Unfortunately, at the current time only 40% of physicians include counseling on physical activity for their patients. A wide variety of resources are available to help physicians who wish to get started or become more knowledgeable in this area. Given the wide range of benefits available to their patients, it is a very important part of comprehensive health care to recommend increased physical activity. In addition, physical activity can confer a wide variety of benefits for physicians themselves and this habit is highly recommended. It will not only yield benefits to physicians but also increase the likelihood that they will counsel in this very important area to their patients.

CLINICAL APPLICATIONS

- Physical activity recommendations should be made by physicians in every clinical encounter.
- A wide variety of resources are available to help physicians make proper physical activity recommendations to their patients.
- Simple steps such as making physical activity a part of the vital signs may help clinicians start the conversation with their patients about increasing physical activity.
- Physicians should emphasize current guidelines for physical activity such as maintaining 30 minutes of moderate or vigorous physical activity on most, if not all, days to accumulate 150 minutes per week as well as two sessions of musculoskeletal exercises per week.

REFERENCES

1. Rippe JM. Lifestyle Medicine (3rd edition). CRC Press (Boca Raton), 2019.
2. 2018 Physical Activity Guidelines Advisory Committee. 2018 Physical Activity Guidelines Advisory Committee Scientific Report. U.S. Department of Health and Human Services (Washington, DC), 2018.
3. Rippe J. Lifestyle Medicine: Deeper, Broader, and More Precise. Am J Lifestyle Med. 2019;13(5):436–439.
4. Exercise is Medicine ® Internet: https://www.exerciseismedicine.org/ [Accessed February 7, 2020].
5. World Health Organization. Interventions on diet and physical activity: what works: evidence tables. 2009.
6. Kennedy M. What physicians need to know, do and say to promote physical activity. Lifestyle Medicine (3rd edition). CRC Press (Boca Raton), 2019.
7. Zoeller R. Physical activity and fitness in the prevention of cardiovascular disease. In Rippe JM. Lifestyle Medicine (3rd edition). CRC Press (Boca Raton), 2019.
8. Rippe J. Lifestyle Medicine. Blackwell Science, Inc. (London), 1999.
9. American College of Lifestyle Medicine. https://www.lifestylemedicine.org/ [Accessed January 28, 2020.]
10. Cohen ML. Changing patterns of infectious disease. Nature. 2000;406(6797): 762–767.
11. Prevention CfDCa. Chronic Disease Overview [Internet]. 2017 [updated June 28, 2017, November 30, 2017]. Available from https://www.cdc.gov/chronicdisease/overview/index.htm.
12. Quality AfHRa. Multiple Chronic Conditions Chartbook: 2010 Medical Expenditure Panel Survey Data. Available from https://www.ahrq.gov/sites/default/files/wysiwyg/professionals/prevention-chronic-care/decision/mcc/mccchartbook.pdf.
13. Bauer U, Briss P, Goodman R, et al. Prevention of chronic disease in the 21st century: elimination of the leading preventable causes of premature death and disability in the USA. The Lancet. 2014;384(9937):45–52.
14. United States Surgeon General and Richmond JB. Healthy People: The Surgeon General's Report on Health Promotion and Disease Prevention. US Government Printing Office (Bethesda, MD), 1979.
15. Healthy People 2020 [Internet]. Washington, DC: U.S. Department of Health and Human Services, Office of Disease Prevention and Health Promotion. https://www.healthypeople.gov/ [Accessed January 6, 2020].

16. Healthy People 2030 [Internet]. Washington, DC: U.S. Department of Health and Human Services, Office of Disease Prevention and Health Promotion. Development of the National Health Promotion and Disease Prevention Objectives for 2030 https://www.healthypeople.gov/2020/About-Healthy-People/Development-Healthy-People-2030. [Accessed January 6, 2020].

17. Bornstein D, Pate R, Pratt M. A review of the national physical activity plans of six countries. J Phys Act Health. 2009;Nov (6):S245–S264.

18. American College of Sports Medicine. https://www.acsm.org/. [Accessed January 28, 2020].

19. Bornstein D, Pate R. From physical activity guidelines to a national activity plan. J Phys Educ Recreat Dance. 2014;85(7):17–22.

20. American Heart Association. https://www.heart.org/. [Accessed January 28, 2020].

21. Stone N, Robinson J, Lichtenstein A, et al. 2013 ACC/AHA guideline on the treatment of blood cholesterol to reduce atherosclerotic cardiovascular risk in adults. A report of the American College of Cardiology/American heart association task force on practice guidelines. Circulation. 2014;129:S1–S45.

22. Phillips E, Kennedy M. The exercise prescription: a tool to improve physical activity. PM&R. 2012;4(11):818–825.

23. Jadczak A, Dollard J, Mahajan N, et al. The perspectives of pre-frail and frail older people on being advised about exercise: a qualitative study. Fam Pract. 2018;35(3):330–335.

24. McLean G, Croteau K, Schofield G. Trust levels of physical activity information sources: a population study. Health Promot J Aust. 2005;16(3):221.

25. Kreuter M, Chheda S, Bull F. How does physician advice influence patient behavior?: Evidence for a priming effect. Arch Fam Med. 2000;9(5):426.

26. O'Brien M, Shields C, Oh P, et al. Health care provider confidence and exercise prescription practices of exercise is medicine Canada workshop attendees. Appl Physiol Nutr Metab. 2016;42(4):384–390.

27. Pinto B, Goldstein M, DePue J, et al. Acceptability and feasibility of physician-based activity counseling: the PAL project. Am J Prev Med. 1998;15(2):95–102.

28. Patricia M. Barnes M, Schoenborn, C. Trends in Adults Receiving a Recommendation for Exercise or Other Physical Activity from a Physician or Other Health Professional 2012. Available from https://www.cdc.gov/nchs/data/databriefs/db86.pdf.

29. Short C, Hayman M, Rebar A, et al. Physical activity recommendations from general practitioners in Australia. Results from a national survey. Aust NZ J Publ Heal. 2016;40(1):83–90.

30. Institute of Medicine. IOM Report: Improving Medical Education—Enhancing the Behavioral and Social Science Content of Medical School Curricula. 2004.

31. Hauer K, Carney P, Chang A, et al. Behavior change counseling curricula for medical trainees: a systematic review. Acad Med. 2012;87(7):956.

32. Dacey M, Kennedy M, Polak R, et al. Physical activity counseling in medical school education: a systematic review. Med Educ Online. 2014;19(1):24325.

33. Lobelo F, de Quevedo IG. The evidence in support of physicians and health care providers as physical activity role models. Am J Lifestyle Med. 2014;1.55982761352012E15.

34. Lifestyle Medicine Education Collaborative. Home. [Internet]. Available from: http://lifestylemedicineeducation.org/.

35. ACSM's Resource Manual for Guidelines for Exercise Testing and Prescription. Wolters Kluwer/Lippincott, Williams & Wilkins, (Philadelphia, PA) 2014.

36. Relationships of moderate-to-vigorous physical activity to all-cause mortality, with highlighted characteristics common to studies of this type. Physical Activity Guidelines Advisory Committee. 2018 Physical Activity Guidelines Advisory Committee Scientific Report. Washington DC: US Department of Health and Human Services; 2018

37. Davis P. Exercise prescription for apparently healthy individuals and for Special populations. In Rippe JM. Lifestyle Medicine (3rd edition). CRC Press (Boca Raton), 2019.
38. American College of Sports Medicine. ACSM Certified Clinical Exercise Physiologist. Internet www.acsm. Org/get-stay-certified/get-certified/cep [Accessed February 7, 2020].
39. Wells K, Lewis C, Leake B, et al. Do physicians preach what they practice?: A study of physicians' health habits and counseling practices. JAMA. 1984;252(20):2846–2848.
40. Olson S, Odo N, Duran A, et al. Burnout and physical activity in Minnesota internal medicine resident physicians. J Grad Med Educ. 2014;6(4):669–674.
41. Montero-Marín J, García-Campayo J, Mera D, et al. A new definition of burnout syndrome based on Farber's proposal. J Occup Med Toxicol. 2009;4(1):31.
42. Shanafelt T, Hasan O, Dyrbye L, et al., editors. Changes in Burnout and Satisfaction with Work-Life Balance in Physicians and the General US Working Population between 2011 and 2014. Mayo Clinic Proceedings; 2015: Elsevier.

13 Exercise Prescription: Practical Applications

KEY POINTS

- The recommended amounts of physical activity from the Physical Activity Guidelines for Americans 2018 Scientific Report include achieving 150 minutes of moderate to vigorous physical activity and two sessions of strength training per week.
- Clinicians should be aware of the various ways that physical activity can be prescribed to every patient.
- The focus of this chapter is to provide learnings that have come from my research organization, Rippe Lifestyle Institute (RLI), which we have developed over the past 25 years of prescribing physical activity to diverse patient and research subjects.

13.1 INTRODUCTION

Throughout this book the importance of regular physical activity as a significant, health promoting habit has been emphasized. There is enormous literature to support this. Most recently, this literature has been summarized in the Physical Activity Guidelines for Americans Scientific Report 2018 (PAGA 2018) (1). The PAGA 2018 document recommends that individuals try to obtain at least 150 minutes of moderate to vigorous physical activity per week as well as two sessions of musculoskeletal strength training. Individuals who have been inactive can start with even much lower levels and still achieve substantial health benefits. The bottom line is that "some activity is better than none."

My research laboratory, RLI, has been prescribing physical activity for individuals for over 25 years. RLI developed much of the background information for the modern walking movement in America (2–6). We have also done extensive work in strength training (7) and weight management (8).

The purpose of the current chapter is to summarize some of the learnings that we have achieved over the past 25 years and also put them in context in specific ways to prescribe physical activity for other physicians and health-care workers.

RLI has also been the leading academic organization in the area of lifestyle medicine. In fact, we coined the term "lifestyle medicine" in the first edition of the textbook that I edited (*Lifestyle Medicine*, Blackwell Science, 1999) (9). This book is now in its third edition, which was published in 2019, and represents the collected wisdom of over 200 individuals who are experts in various aspects of lifestyle medicine (10). Thus, for physicians and other health-care workers there is an important opportunity to put physical activity in the framework of these lifestyle medicine practices and habits that we should be recommending to all of our patients.

13.2 PRE-PARTICIPATION SCREENING

A key concept underscored in the Physical Activity Guidelines for Americans 2008 (11) and reiterated in the PAGA Committee Scientific Report 2018 is that when it comes to physical activity "some is better than none." With this in mind, both the American College of Sports Medicine (ACSM) (12) and the PAGA 2018 recommend that clinicians have a discussion with every patient and make it as easy as possible for individuals to become more physically active. This is particularly true for individuals who have been very inactive.

To get this started, the first order of pre-participation screening is simply to inquire from individuals how much physical activity they do and then begin to work with them to increase the physical activity. It can be noted that the recommended guidelines by the PAGA 2018 is to accumulate 150 minutes of moderate to vigorous activity on a weekly basis and, in addition, two strength training sessions. It should be emphasized, however, that for inactive individuals even 30 minutes per week is sufficient to yield significant reduction in risk both of all-cause mortality and specifically mortality from cardiovascular disease (CVD) (13).

One good way of starting the conversation about the level of physical activity is to use the recommendation incorporated by both the U.S. National Physical Activity Program (14) and the Exercise is Medicine initiative (15). This involves utilizing a tool consisting of two questions which was developed at Stanford University:

- On average, how many days a week do you engage in moderate or strenuous physical activity (like a brisk walk)?
- On average, how many minutes do you engage in exercise at this level?

Answers to these questions should give the clinician a good place to start to help individuals gradually increase their physical activity, if necessary, with the goal to ultimately meet the guidelines from the PAGA 2018 Scientific Report.

The next level of pre-participation screening could involve a brief questionnaire called the "PAR Q" (16). This stands for "Physical Activity Readiness Questionnaire" and is found in Appendix A. Both of these questionnaires can assist in determining what level of physical activity prescription to make and also whether or not there are any further tests required.

Other tests are also available to estimate where a person should start on a physical activity program. One that we developed at my research laboratory, RLI, is the One-mile Walk Test (3). This is a relatively easy test to take. However, it may be more than the inactive person needs to get started. It simply involves walking a mile at a brisk pace, taking a heart rate at the end of the mile, then utilizing a table based on these parameters as well as gender and age to estimate aerobic fitness (VO_2 Max). More detail about how to take the One-mile Walk Test may be found in Appendix B.

13.3   PRINCIPLES OF EXERCISE PRESCRIPTION

It is important to emphasize that the key for sedentary individuals is simply to get more activity in their lives. Thus, the typical way that exercise is prescribed by exercise physiologists and the principles endorsed by organizations such as ACSM (17, 18) are typically not necessary for individuals who have been sedentary and simply want to incorporate more physical activity in their lives.

If a clinician wants to be more precise in terms of the exercise and physical activity prescription, the framework recommended by the ACSM (17, 18) goes by the acronym "FITT" can be utilized. This stands for the following:

- Frequency
- Intensity
- Time
- Type

Typically, a *frequency* of three or more times a week of moderate to vigorous physical activity is recommended. *Intensity* is typically recommended to be at 50–70% of predicted maximum heart rate or at a perceived exertion that is considered to be "moderate." (A good way of thinking about this level of intensity is that if you are walking, the pace should be more than simply ambling, such as you might do when you are shopping, but it is not racewalking.) Typical speeds for most people for this type of walking are 3.5 to 4 miles per hour or what would be considered as a "brisk walk." President Harry Truman was famous for providing what is essentially a way of thinking about brisk walking, when he told the Secret Service Men who tried to keep up with him on one of his daily walks is that they should "walk as though you have someplace to go."

Time denotes the number of minutes that the individual is involved in physical activity. The classic way of thinking about "time" comes from ACSM with the recommendation of 30 minutes per session. The 2008 PAGA recommended breaking physical activity into sessions of 10 minutes or more to yield health benefits, whereas the PAGA 2018 documented that sessions even shorter than 10 minutes accumulated throughout the day also yielded health benefits.

Type involves what type of physical activity is performed. For greater than 90% of individuals the physicians see this will involve walking. The area of walking has been something where my research laboratory has been a leading research and program provider for many years (2–6). More about this will be discussed in the next section.

13.4   AEROBIC PHYSICAL ACTIVITY/EXERCISE PRESCRIPTION

Aerobic activities are typically defined as those that require oxygen to provide energy. These activities typically involve large muscle groups used in a repeated or rhythmic fashion. Other forms of physical activity can certainly be included in aerobic activity; however, walking is one of the most popular forms of this type of physical activity.

Recent advances in technology have given us the ability to prescribe physical activity with more precision than that was prescribed in the past. These technologies, however, are not essential if the goal is simply to get sedentary individuals to increase their amount of regular aerobic activity. The PAGA 2018 Scientific Report recommends that people participate in 150 minutes of aerobic physical activity per week (1). Individuals who have been quite sedentary in the past may find this difficult to achieve and should work up to this slowly.

- *Walking*—Walking is by far the most popular form of regular physical activity. When physicians are surveyed concerning the type of physical activity they would recommend for their patients, over 90% say "walking."

    My laboratory and clinic, RLI, has been a leading source of walking research for the past 25 years. In fact, we coined the term "fitness walking" with the publication of our first book of that name in this area, back in the early 1980s (19). We also developed the first "field" test of walking (the One-mile Walk Test), which enables individuals to assess their level of fitness by taking this simple test (3).

    There are multiple benefits for walking. It is, as a practical matter, one of the most convenient and easy forms of aerobic physical activity. Walking does not require any specialized equipment (except for potentially a good pair of walking or running shoes). In addition, walking is an activity that virtually everyone is familiar with and has the added benefit of being low impact, since one foot is always in touch with the ground. Walking involves only 1–1.5 times an individual's body weight on each stride. In comparison, running generates over three times a person's body weight each time his/her foot lands.

    Activities such as basketball can generate forces up to six times body weight when landing. Low impact (4) is very important for individuals who have been sedentary and might risk injury or joint discomfort involving more vigorous activity such as running. Low impact is also very important for individuals who are overweight or obese since the forces are compounded due to the extra weight.

    The walking programs my research team has developed are found in Appendix B.

    These walking programs range all the way from ones appropriate for sedentary individuals to ones for individuals who are quite fit. We use the color spectrum to indicate the different programs. The blue program is defined for individuals who are the least fit, while the green, yellow, orange, and red programs are progressively more vigorous.

    In each of these programs we recommend a specific pace and distance, a recommended warm-up and cooldown as well as frequency. As the concept of "steps" has become more popular in the area of physical activity, we have now included in these programs how many steps per day we are recommending. Thus, individuals can utilize either steps or distance to monitor their walking program.

Of course, many of the technological fitness devices that are now available also contain GPS systems; so both steps and distance are typically available, if an individual has one of these technologies such as an Apple wristwatch or activity monitor. (Fit Bit on equivalent.)

- *Other forms of aerobic activity*—There are many other excellent forms of aerobic activity in addition to, or as a substitute or in combination with, walking. For example, stationary cycling or swimming are also excellent forms of aerobic activity and have low impact. If your patients prefer to utilize one of the other types of aerobic activities rather than walking, simply use the walking protocols found in Appendix B, but utilize the same number of minutes each week as outlined in the walking programs and the same level of intensity. The walking programs vary from 20 to 40 minutes in length and these should be the guidelines for other forms of aerobic activities as well.

13.5   MUSCULAR FITNESS

Muscular fitness is important for a variety of reasons including the ability to perform the activities of daily living as well as maintaining balance and performing various fitness activities with lower risk of injuries. The two components of muscular fitness are interrelated. One is muscular strength, which is the maximum amount of force a muscle group can produce (17, 18). Strength is what is typically utilized in single effort activities such as moving a heavy box, lifting a heavy bag of groceries, and lifting a young child or grandchild. Muscular endurance is the ability of a muscle or muscle group to exert force repeatedly over time or maintain a contraction over a period of time. Both components of muscular fitness are important.

In addition, muscular fitness is very important to lower the age-related loss of muscle. Individuals typically lose muscle progressively after the age of 40. This can result in about a 1% loss of muscle per year and accelerate to the point where there is a 10–15% loss of lean muscle per decade, particularly over the age of 60 (20). Muscle loss can not only lower strength and endurance but also slow metabolism. Muscular fitness has also been shown in multiple studies to contribute to lowering the risk of various metabolic conditions such as heart disease and diabetes.

For all of these reasons, the PAGA Scientific Report 2018 and the ACSM recommend two muscular fitness sessions per week. These sessions should be separated by at least one day. In my research laboratory at RLI, we typically include strength training as a component of an overall fitness program.

There are several important considerations if you are going to recommend a strength training program for your patients. First, it is imperative that an individual who is not previously experienced in muscular strength training seek professional guidance that may be available from a fitness trainer at a health club or YMCA. The highest level of fitness trainers also carry a fitness training certification from ACSM. Clinicians should inquire about this certification before referring patients to a trainer.

Second, it is important to include exercises that involve all of the major muscle groups. These include the following:

- Quadriceps (front of thighs)
- Hamstring (back of thighs)
- Hips
- Abdomen
- Biceps
- Triceps
- Chest

It is also important to emphasize to your patients that a 5–7 minute warm-up and cooldown will help avoid injuries and lower the amount of muscle soreness after strength training.

Progression should be slow as in aerobic exercises. As a practical matter, strength training can occur with exercise machines, such as at a fitness club, free weights or elastic bands, or using the individual's own body weight (e.g. push-ups, sit-ups). There are multiple programs that can be done both at fitness facilities and also at home. One home program that we developed at RLI for strength training may be found in Appendix C. Strength training programs should be performed two or three times a week with at least one day off between sessions.

13.6   FLEXIBILITY

Flexibility is the ability of a joint to move through its full range of motion. Flexibility is an important part of an overall, comprehensive program of physical activity. It allows not only other forms of physical activity, but also activities of daily living to be performed with reduced risk of injury. Flexibility is particularly important since disuse or aging can lower this parameter. At RLI, we typically recommend flexibility programs for all of the individuals that we see either in our clinic or in our research trials. Flexibility is also considered an important part of a comprehensive exercise program by both ACSM and the PAGA Scientific Report 2018. Engaging in flexibility exercises during warm-up and cooldown will allow your patients to have some benefits of mind/body relaxation techniques.

The flexibility exercises we employ for patients or research subjects at RLI typically are part of the 5–7 minutes warm-up and 5–7 minutes cooldown. Stretching should occur both before and after every session of physical activity. If you want to recommend to your patients that they derive a baseline test of their current flexibility, one good and easy to perform test is called the "Sit and Reach Test." We often utilize this test to provide background information to individuals in our research programs. It can also be viewed simply by Googling "Sit and Reach Test."

There are two good ways to engage in regular stretching. One is called "Static" stretching. This is the most common method to improve flexibility and involves slowly moving a joint to the point where you begin to feel tension in the muscle being stretched and then holding that position for 10–30 seconds. It is important not to place the joint in any position that actually causes pain. The other type of flexibility exercise is called "Dynamic" stretching. This type of stretching involves moving parts of your body through a full range of motion, while gradually increasing the reach and speed of the movement in a controlled manner. A good example of this would be arm circles, where you begin with small circles and then gradually progress to larger and faster circles. One caution is not to perform what is called "Ballistic" stretching, where a person bounces up and down in a stretch. This may actually cause injury.

There are a variety of programs available for stretching. These may be found in any of the books put out by ACSM. One book I can recommend for general advice about flexibility and other aspects of fitness is the *American College of Sports Medicine Complete Guide to Fitness and Health* edited by Dr Barbara Bushman (18). This is available through Human Kinetics press.

13.7 DURATION OF WORKOUTS

For many years, it was thought that the duration of a bout of physical activity needed to at least ten minutes in order to yield important health benefits. In fact, this is what was incorporated in the guidance from the ACSM (21). I was pleased to have been one of the co-authors of this recommendation that was incorporated into the 2008 Physical Activity Guidelines for Americans. In the ensuing decade between 2008 and 2018, abundant new information became available indicating that physical activity sessions of less than ten minutes per session could also result in significant health and fitness benefits. For this reason, the PAGA 2018 Scientific Report recommended that any duration of physical activity could yield important benefits. This is particularly important to emphasize to your patients who have been sedentary. You should counsel sedentary patients that even small amounts of regular physical activity such as taking the stairs at work or parking further away from stores and walking across the parking lot when shopping, if done on a regular basis, can yield important health and fitness benefits. Thus, the barrier of needing to get physical activity in sessions of ten minutes or more has now been essentially removed.

Physicians should encourage inactive individuals to recognize that getting even small amounts of physical activity can result in important health and fitness benefits. Remember the mantra "some is better than none."

13.8 BALANCE

Balance is a very important part of an overall plan for physical activity. This should be a component of an exercise prescription, particularly for older individuals. Improving balance can occur either with specific balance exercises or by increasing physical activity and muscular fitness.

There are a number of balance tests available. Some are very simple and can be conducted at home. The one that we have used in a number of our research trials is the "Single Leg Stand Test", which involves how long an individual can maintain balance standing on one foot at a time. This can occur initially with eyes open and then, subsequently, with eyes closed. Details about how to conduct this test are, once again, available through multiple ACSM publications. The PAGA Scientific Report 2018 recommends a variety of balance tests and incorporates this component as part of a comprehensive program of physical activity.

13.9   MIND/BODY APPROACHES

Increased physical activity is also a great time to practice mind/body modalities, recognizing that the mind and body are intimately connected. This is particularly important in an era where enormous stress is prevalent among people. Many of the mind/body techniques involve gentle forms of exercises. For example, both yoga and Tai Chi incorporate not only physical activity movements but also ways of incorporating mind/body meditation. The "relaxation response" popularized by Dr Herb Benson is also a technique that can be employed while walking because the rhythmic motion of walking can lend itself to focusing on mind/body interactions (22).

The connections between mind and body are a very powerful way of helping people understand how multiple health and fitness domains can be benefitted by increased physical activity. It should also be noted that regular physical activity is a very powerful stress reducer. In fact, many regular exercisers indicate that stress reduction is a major reason why they are engaged in regular physical activity. There are also good data to suggest that regular physical activity lowers both depression and anxiety, which are important components of stress. (See Chapter 11 for more details.)

We routinely recommend to individuals that they use the warm-up and cooldown portions of their physical activity program as a time when they can not only stretch their joints and muscles but also engage in mindful meditation, which will enhance the pleasure and benefit of their physical activity session and reduce stress.

13.10   EXERCISE ADHERENCE

While a number of physical activity benefits accrue immediately following each session, most of the health and fitness benefits including reduction of risk of chronic disease accrue to individuals who stay with their exercise program throughout a lifetime. For this reason, it is important to emphasize to your patients that adhering to an exercise program is very important.

It is also important to identify potential barriers to continuing an exercise program and help your patients understand these potential barriers and plan to overcome them. One important aspect of exercise adherence is to find the type of exercise that an individual finds both enjoyable and easy to perform. Another key component is finding a physical activity program that has a low injury potential. Some of these factors apply to the individual. Other factors include the availability of physical activity facilities such as walking paths, health clubs, or YMCAs.

It is important to emphasize the long-term benefits of physical activity to your patients at every clinic visit, which will help an individual understand that there are multiple benefits from sticking with their exercise program.

13.11   SPECIAL POPULATIONS

A variety of special populations should be considered when recommendations for physical activity are given. For public health considerations, the population is typically divided by age group into youth, adult, and older adults. These are the definitions that are utilized in this book. There are separate chapters on physical activity in each of these populations. (See Chapters 1, 7, and 8.) As a general statement, the PAGA 2018 Scientific Report recommends that youth should be encouraged to devote 60 minutes each day to moderate to vigorous physical activity. Older adults have the same general recommendation of 150 minutes of moderate to vigorous physical activity on a weekly basis, as do adults between the ages of 18 and 65. The intensity level in older adults, however, may need to be somewhat decreased due to lower fitness capacity for individuals as they age.

Other special populations include women following pregnancy (this is handled in Chapter 6) and individuals with various chronic conditions (these recommendations are handled in Chapter 9). The general recommendation of 150 minutes of moderate to vigorous physical activity still applies to most of these special populations, although special considerations may need to be given to any specific conditions that may modify the type of physical activity or duration. Recommendations for individuals who are cancer survivors (Chapter 4) and who have heart disease (Chapter 3) or diabetes (Chapter 5) are all handled in separate chapters.

The bottom-line message for virtually every individual, even if they are in a special population, is that increased physical activity yields multiple short-term and long-term benefits. Thus, virtually every individual seen in clinical practice should have a discussion of physical activity and recommendations made to increase it if they are below the guidelines for the PAGA 2018 Scientific Report of 150 minutes of moderate to vigorous physical activity on a weekly basis and two strength training sessions per week.

13.12   TIPS FOR STARTING AND STAYING WITH A PROGRAM OF REGULAR PHYSICAL ACTIVITY

Over the past 25 years, my team at RLI has had the opportunity to recommend physical activity to thousands of patients and research subjects. Over that period of time we have developed a variety of tips to help people get started and stay with a regular physical activity program. Many of these tips were developed with our walking research and clinical programs, but they equally apply to any program of physical activity. Here are some tips that we have developed that can be utilized by clinicians to help their patients start and stay with physical activity program (4):

- *Exercise with others*—Having other individuals to exercise with can make it into a more enjoyable social experience. This may involve taking group exercise classes at a fitness facility or simply finding friends to exercise with.
- *Establish a time and place*—Make physical activity a priority. If you leave your physical activity program as a nebulous part of your life and do not establish a specific time and place within your calendar to block off for physical activity, it is less likely that you will participate in it.
- *Find an activity you enjoy*—Having an enjoyable experience in physical activity is a key to looking forward to it every day.

- *Keep a journal*—Writing down your progress is a habit that many regular exercisers have adopted throughout their life. Journaling allows you to see how much progress that you have made and also note parts of your physical activity program that you want to remember.
- *Elicit the support of family and friends*—Having other people who care about you know that you are working on your health through a physical activity program can be very motivational.
- *Set realistic goals*—Many times people falter by choosing the wrong type of physical activity or engaging in too much right away or progressing too rapidly. This applies to walking or running programs or any other type of physical activity.
- *Purchase appropriate equipment*—This may be as simple as getting a good pair of walking shoes and also all-weather gear if you are going to walk or run outside. Other forms of physical activity are made more enjoyable if you have the right equipment. For example, in swimming get a good swimsuit and a pair of good goggles that do not leak water.
- *Vary your exercise routines*—In walking this may be accomplished by taking different walking routes or by blending different types of physical activities such as walking three times a week and stationary cycling three times a week.
- *Avoid injury*—The key to avoiding injury is to choose the types of activities that are lowest in injury potential such as walking, swimming, or stationary cycling and also not progressing too rapidly, which can lead to injuries and excessive soreness.
- *Upgrade your fitness program as you progress*—As you continue on with your physical activity program, be sure to have slow progression so that you gain all the benefits of increased physical activity. For individuals who have been very sedentary in the past, even small amounts of physical activity can yield enormous benefits, but ultimately the goal is to slowly progress to the recommended 150 minutes of moderate or vigorous physical activity per week.
- *Reward yourself*—By choosing to be more physically active you have made one of the most important health-related decisions possible in your life. Allow yourself to celebrate and reward your progress and your commitment. Not only are you improving your health and lowering your risk of chronic disease, but you are also improving your mental outlook and building more endurance. You will also simply look and feel better by engaging in regular physical activity.

13.13 CONCLUSIONS

Prescribing regular physical activity is one of the key considerations that every clinician can and should do for every patient. As indicated throughout this book, there are enormous benefits from a physically active lifestyle and enormous health risks for people who are inactive. It does not take a lot of physical activity to yield significant health benefits. We also know that physician recommendation is one of the most powerful motivators for people to participate in physical activity. Unfortunately, only about 40% of physicians are regularly recommending physical activity. By following some of the recommendations in this chapter you can help guide your patients to a more physically active lifestyle and help them achieve the multiple health benefits that are derived from regular physical activity.

CLINICAL APPLICATIONS

- Increased physical activity will yield multiple benefits for virtually every patient.
- Comprehensive physical activity should include aerobic activity and muscular fitness, and may also include flexibility, balance, and mind/body considerations.
- Clinicians should become knowledgeable about ways that they can motivate their patients to include more physical activity in their daily lives and derive the multiple health benefits from this habit.

REFERENCES

1. 2018 Physical Activity Guidelines Advisory Committee. 2018 Physical Activity Guidelines Advisory Committee Scientific Report. U.S. Department of Health and Human Services (Washington, DC), 2018.
2. Rippe J, Ward A, Porcari J, et al. Walking for health and fitness. JAMA. 1988;259:272.
3. Kline G, Porcari J, Hintermeister R, et al. Estimation of VO_2 max from a one-mile track walk, gender, age, and body weight. Med Sci Sports Exerc. 1987;19:253–259.
4. Rippe J, Ward A. The Complete Book of Fitness Walking. Prentice Hall Press (New York), 1990.
5. Rippe J, Ward A. The Rockport Walking Program. Prentice Hall Press (New York), 1989.
6. Kashiwa A, Rippe J. Fitness Walking for Women. Putnam (New York), 1987.
7. Rippe J. The Exercise Exchange Program. Simon & Schuster (New York), 1992.
8. Rippe J, Angelopoulos T. Obesity: Prevention and Treatment. CRC Press (Boca Raton), 2012.
9. Rippe J. Lifestyle Medicine. Blackwell Science, Inc. (London), 1999.
10. Rippe J. Lifestyle Medicine (3rd edition). CRC Press (Boca Raton), 2019.
11. 2008 Physical Activity Guidelines Advisory Committee. 2018 Physical Activity Guidelines Advisory Committee Scientific Report. U.S. Department of Health and Human Services (Washington, DC), 2008.
12. Napolitano M, Lewis B, Whiteley J, et al. Theoretical foundations of physical activity behavior change. ACSM's Resource Manual for Guidelines for Exercise Testing and Prescription (7th edition). Lippincott, Williams & Wilkins (New York, NY). 2013;730–744.
13. Moore S, Patel A, Matthews C. Leisure time physical activity of moderate to vigorous intensity and mortality: a large pooled cohort analysis. PLoS Med. 2012;9(11).
14. Bornstein D, Pate R. From physical activity guidelines to a national activity plan. J Phys Educ Recreat Dance. 2014;85(7):17–22.
15. Medicine ACos. Exercise is Medicine. Available from http//exerciseismedicine.org/.
16. Warburton D, Jamnik V, Bredin S, et al. PAR-Q+ research collaboration. The physical activity readiness questionnaire (PAR-Q+) and electronic physical activity readiness medical examination (ePARmed-X+). Health Fitness J Can. 2011;4(2):3–23.

17. ACSM's Resource Manual for Guidelines for Exercise Testing and Prescription (7th edition). Wolters Kluwer/Lippincott Williams & Wilkins (Philadelphia, PA), 2014.
18. Bushman B. American College of Sports Medicine Complete Guide to Fitness Health (2nd edition). Human Kinetics (Champaign, IL), 2017.
19. Sweetgall R, Rippe J, Katch F. Fitness Walking. Putnam (New York), 1985.
20. Leon A. Reducing aging-associated risk of sarcopenia. In Rippe JM. Lifestyle Medicine (3rd edition). CRC Press (Boca Raton), 2019.
21. Pate R, Pratt M, Blair S, et al. Physical activity and public health: a recommendation from the centers for disease control and prevention and the American College of sports medicine. JAMA. 1995;273:402–407.
22. Benson H. The Relaxation Response. William Morrow and Co, Inc. (New York, NY), 1975.

14 Overcoming Sedentary Behavior

KEY POINTS

- Sedentary behavior, particularly at high levels (more than seven hours of sitting or lying down during waking hours per day), is associated with increased risk of all-cause mortality and mortality from cardiovascular disease and Type 2 diabetes, as well as some cancers.
- Regular, moderate to vigorous physical activity can offset many of the increased risks associated with sedentary behavior.
- Benefits of moderate to vigorous physical activity are particularly strong for individuals with high levels of sedentary behavior and who are currently inactive.

14.1 INTRODUCTION

Considerable research has emerged over the past decade in the area of sedentary behavior (1). Good data are now available to suggest that sedentary behavior increases the risk of a variety of conditions including coronary heart disease (CHD) and Type 2diabetes (T2DM). Sedentary behavior is defined as "any behavior which is characterized by an energy expenditure of 1.5 METs or less, while in a sitting, reclining, or lying posture (2)."

In addition to its negative association with health outcomes, sedentary behavior is highly prevalent in the United Statespopulation. Data from the U.S. National Health and Nutrition Examination Survey (NHANES) indicate that children and adults in the US spend approximately 7.7 hours per day (55% of monitored time) being sedentary (3). Thus, reversing this sedentary behavior trend in the United Statescould generate significant health improvements. The current chapter examines sedentary behavior and its relationship to various health issues using the framework established by the Physical Activity Guidelines for Americans 2018 Advisory Committee Scientific Report (1).

14.2 SEDENTARY BEHAVIOR AND ALL-CAUSE MORTALITY

The PAGA 2018 Scientific Report rated the evidence for a relationship between the greater amount of time in sedentary behavior and all-cause mortality as strong (1). Based on a total of nine systematic reviews and meta-analyses that consisted of twenty original studies, a significant relationship between sedentary behavior and all-cause mortality was revealed (4–11). In addition, some of the studies showed that TV viewing or screen time were also related to all-cause mortality (12, 13). There also appears to be a dose-response relationship between sedentary behavior and all-cause mortality (7, 9). The studies that have been reviewed showed that for every one hour increase in sitting time, or for more than seven hours a day sitting, there were dose-related responses to increased sedentary behavior and all-cause mortality (7). A similar response was revealed between TV viewing and all-cause mortality where, once again, using different criteria, a dose-response relationship was found (9).

An inverse relationship exists between the amount of moderate to vigorous physical activity and sedentary behavior when it comes to all-cause mortality (10, 11). The adverse effects on all-cause mortality from sedentary behavior are strongest amongst people who have low amounts of physical activity. This relationship is illustrated in Figure 14.1.

Individuals who were found to have greater than seven hours of sedentary behavior and also low levels of moderate to vigorous physical activity substantially increased their risk of all-cause mortality. Individuals who accumulated between 16 and 30 MET hours per week of moderate intensity physical activity substantially lowered their risk of all-cause mortality, even if they were sedentary for more than seven hours per day (11).

To put this in perspective, the PAGA 2018 recommends between 10 and 15 MET hours per week of physical activity. There are additional benefits for individuals

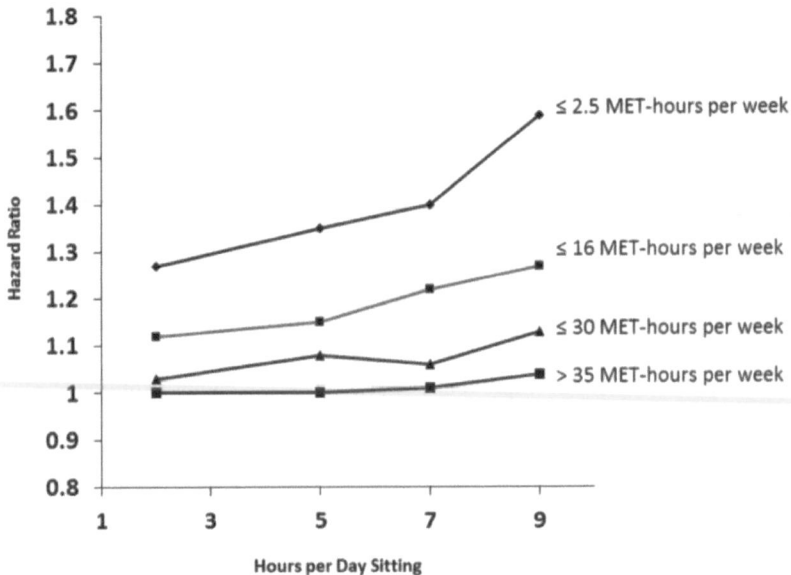

FIGURE 14.1   Relationship between sitting and all-cause mortality, stratified by amount of moderate-to-vigorous physical activity.

(Adapted from data found in Ekelund et al. 2016. 2018 Physical Activity Guidelines Advisory Committee. 2018 Physical Activity Committee Scientific Report. Washington, DC US Department of Health and Human Services; 2018. Part F, Chapter 2, Sedentary Behavior.)

who achieve greater than 30 MET hours per week, although the incremental benefit is relatively small compared to the benefit of meeting the recommended dosage of moderate to vigorous physical activity outlined in the PAGA 2018 document. Individuals who have sedentary occupations (such as office work), thus, will particularly benefit from following the guidelines for moderate to vigorous physical activity on a weekly basis.

There has also been some suggestion that taking breaks in sedentary behavior may reduce its adverse health effects related to all-cause mortality. Some research exists in this area, although further research is required to determine whether or not periodic breaks in sedentary behavior will ameliorate some of the adverse health effects of high levels of this behavior.

The relationship between sedentary time and moderate to vigorous physical activity is depicted graphically in Figure 14.2 (1).

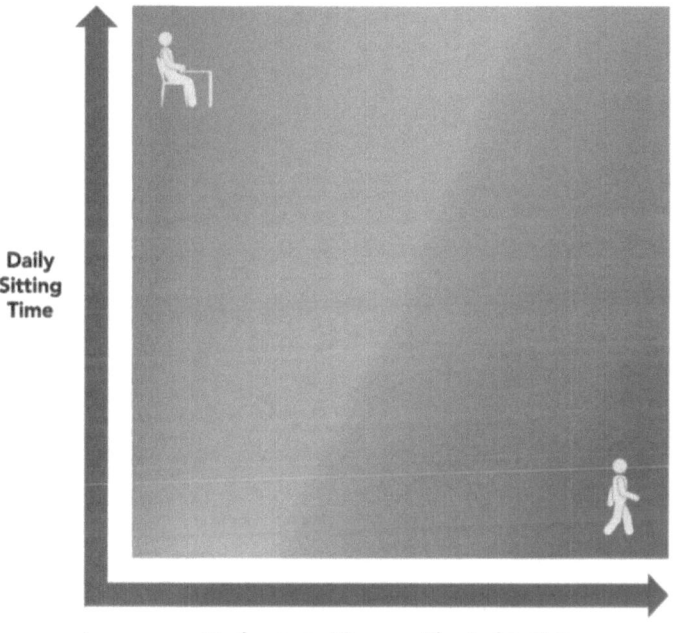

Daily Sitting Time

Moderate-to-Vigorous Physical Activity

Risk of all-cause mortality decreases as one moves from gray to black.

FIGURE 14.2   Relationship among moderate-to-vigorous physical activity, sitting time, and risk of all-cause mortality.

(Adapted from data found in Ekelund et al. 2016. 2018 Physical Activity Guidelines Advisory Committee. 2018 Physical Activity Committee Scientific Report. Washington, DC US Department of Health and Human Services; 2018. Part F, Chapter 2, Sedentary Behavior.)

As this figure shows, the more sedentary time an individual participates in, the more the risk of all-cause mortality, unless they are physically active. Physical activity, as shown in this figure, largely can ameliorate the increased risk of sedentary behavior.

14.3 SEDENTARY BEHAVIOR AND CARDIOVASCULAR DISEASE MORTALITY

The risk of mortality from cardiovascular disease (CVD) and its relationship to sedentary behavior is very similar to the relationship between sedentary behavior and all-cause mortality (6, 10). The PAGA 2018 Scientific Report documented that increased physical activity of ameliorated increases in sedentary behavior. In addition, there was strong evidence that there was a dose-response relationship. Thus, the more physical activity an individual participates in, the more the increased risk of sedentary behavior is reduced. As depicted in Figure 14.3 sedentary behavior of greater than five hours a day starts to significantly increase the risk of cardiovascular disease and it is further increased if sedentary behavior is greater than seven hours per day (1).

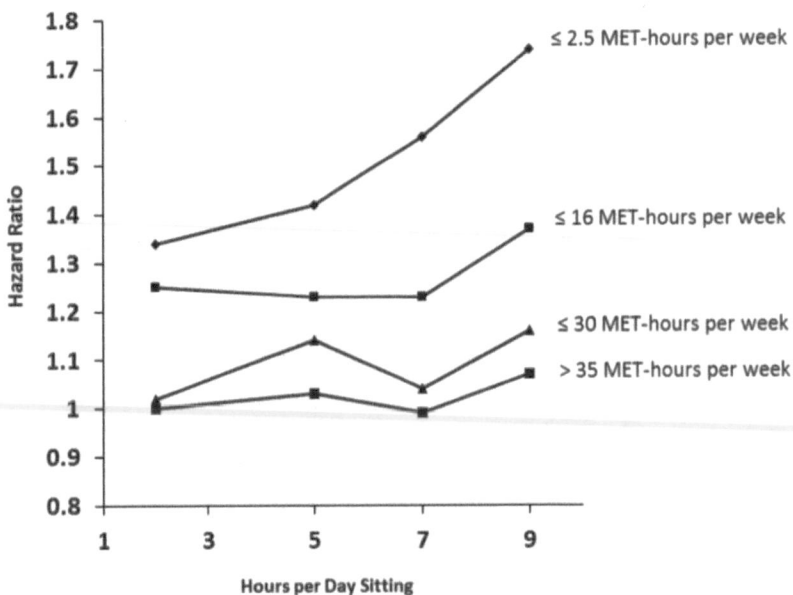

FIGURE 14.3 Relationship between sitting and cardiovascular disease mortality, stratified by amount of moderate-to-vigorous physical activity.

(Adapted from data found in Ekelund et al. 2016. 2018 Physical Activity Guidelines Advisory Committee. 2018 Physical Activity Committee Scientific Report. Washington, DC US Department of Health and Human Services; 2018. Part F, Chapter 2, Sedentary Behavior).

14.4   SEDENTARY BEHAVIOR AND CANCER MORTALITY

The PAGA 2018 Scientific Report judged the evidence between a direct relationship with the amount of time spent in sedentary behavior and higher mortality rates from cancer as limited (10). While a number of studies have reported a significant association, the results were inconsistent. (One study showed a relationship for women only; another one showed one only for television viewing, but not sitting; and one showed a relationship only in current smokers.) Furthermore, cancer is a heterogeneous disease and many of the risk factors for cancer mortality are clearly affected by cancer screening, treatment availability, and efficacy.

The PAGA 2018 Scientific Report also concluded that there was insufficient evidence available to determine whether or not the relationship between sedentary behavior and cancer mortality was modified by physical activity. Evidence among specific types of cancer was moderate (14). For example, moderate level physical activity in sedentary individuals was related to decrease in added risk for breast cancer, ovarian cancer, prostate cancer, and lung cancer.

14.5   SEDENTARY BEHAVIOR AND TYPE 2 DIABETES

There is strong evidence that a significant relationship exists between the amount of time spent in sedentary behavior and risk of Type 2 diabetes (T2DM) (4–6, 10, 13). The issue of whether or not there is a dose-response relationship, however, is only supported by limited evidence. The issue of TV viewing appeared to be different between individuals who were active and inactive. Active individuals did not experience elevated risk of T2DM, whereas, inactive participants who reported high TV viewing were at increased risk for Type 2 diabetes (T2DM). More detail about physical activity and T2 DM may be found in Chapter 5.

14.6   SEDENTARY BEHAVIOR AND WEIGHT STATUS

Limited evidence supports a relationship between sedentary behavior and weight status (4, 5). The studies that are available in this area showed considerable variations among results. With regard to adiposity, once again studies are quite heterogeneous, allowing only limited support for the concept that sedentary behavior is associated with adiposity.

14.7   SEDENTARY BEHAVIOR AND MODERATE TO VIGOROUS PHYSICAL ACTIVITY

There is some evidence that moderate to vigorous physical activity lowers the risk of sedentary behavior (11). It is important to note, however, that the relative reductions in risk are most significant for those who are the most sedentary. In general, the same relationship holds for CVD mortality as well as for all-cause mortality with significant interaction between level of physical activity and sedentary behavior. Again, the most significant benefits come to those who are the most sedentary. When the data concerning sedentary behavior are stratified by level of sitting or TV viewing, the relationships are still quite similar with the amount of sedentary behavior, sitting or TV viewing significantly increasing the risk of all-cause mortality, while the level of moderate to vigorous physical activity lowers the added risk in a dose-response manner.

14.8   PUBLIC HEALTH IMPACT

High levels of sedentary behavior are associated with increases in all-cause mortality, mortality from CVD and T2DM. High levels of sedentary behavior are also associated with moderate increases in certain cancers such as those of breast, ovary, and prostate.

There is good evidence that moderate or vigorous physical activity can lower the increased risk associated with sedentary behavior. This is particularly striking in individuals who have the highest level of sedentary behavior. For all of these reasons, physicians should assess the level of sedentary behavior in every patient and, if needed, recommend increased levels of moderate to vigorous physical activity. The public health impact on such changes could be very significant.

14.9   CONCLUSIONS

Both children and adults in the United Stateshave become increasingly sedentary. The average child or adult in the United States spends 7.7 hours per day being sedentary. This includes screen time, watching TV, and other tasks sitting or lying down. These levels of sedentary behavior have now been clearly demonstrated to increase all-cause mortality and mortality from CVD, T2DM, and some cancers. Levels of moderate to vigorous physical activity can offset the increased risk of sedentary behavior. This is particularly true for individuals who have the highest levels of sedentary behavior and are also inactive. For all of these reasons, physicians should assess the level of sedentary behavior in every patient and, if necessary, recommend increased levels of moderate to vigorous physical activity to lower the increased risk of sedentary behavior.

CLINICAL APPLICATIONS

- Sedentary behavior, particularly at levels of greater than seven hours per day, is associated with increased risk of all-cause mortality.
- Sedentary behavior is also associated with increased risk of CVD and T2DM as well as some cancers.
- Moderate to vigorous physical activity may offset the adverse consequences of sedentary behavior, particularly in individuals who have high levels of sedentary behavior and are also currently inactive.
- Physicians should assess levels of sedentary behavior in every patient and recommend increased levels of moderate or vigorous physical activity, if necessary.

REFERENCES

1. 2018 Physical Activity Guidelines Advisory Committee. 2018 Physical Activity Guidelines Advisory Committee Scientific Report. Washington, DC: U.S. Department of Health and Human Services, 2018. Part F. Chapter 2. Sedentary Behavior.
2. Tremblay M, Aubert S, Barnes J, et al. SBRN terminology consensus project participants. Int J Behav Nutr Phys Act. 2017;14(1):75.

3. Matthews C, Chen K, Freedson P, et al. Amount of time spent in sedentary behaviors in the United States, 2003-2004. Am J Epidemiol. 2008;167(7):875–881.

4. Proper K, Singh A, van Mechelen W, et al. Sedentary behaviors and health outcomes among adults: a systematic review of prospective studies. Am J Prev Med. 2011;40(2):174–182.

5. Thorp A, Owen N, Neuhaus M, et al. Sedentary behaviors and subsequent health outcomes in adults a systematic review of longitudinal studies, 1996–2011. Am J Prev Med. 2011;41(2):207–215.

6. Wilmot E, Edwardson C, Achana F, et al. Sedentary time in adults and the association with diabetes, cardiovascular disease and death: systematic review and meta-analysis. Diabetologia. 2012;55(11):2895–2905.

7. Chau J, Grunseit A, Chey T, et al. Daily sitting time and all-cause mortality: a meta-analysis. PLoS One. 2013;8(11):e80000.

8. de Rezende L, Rey-Lopez J, Matsudo V, et al. Sedentary behavior and health outcomes among older adults: a systematic review. BMC Public Health. 2014;14:333. doi:10.1186/1471- 2458-14-333.

9. Sun J, Zhao L, Yang Y, et al. Association between television viewing time and all-cause mortality: a meta-analysis of cohort studies. Am J Epidemiol. 2015;182(11):908–16.

10. Biswas A, Oh P, Faulkner G, et al. Sedentary time and its association with risk for disease incidence, mortality, and hospitalization in adults: a systematic review and meta-analysis. Ann Intern Med. 2015;162(2):123–132.

11. Ekelund U, Steene-Johannessen J, Brown W, et al. Does physical activity attenuate, or even eliminate, the detrimental association of sitting time with mortality? A harmonised meta-analysis of data from more than 1 million men and women. Lancet. 2016;388(10051):1302–1310.

12. George S, Smith A, Alfano C, et al. The association between television watching time and allcause mortality after breast cancer. J Cancer Surviv. 2013;7(2):247–252.

13. Grontved A, Hu F. Television viewing and risk of type 2 diabetes, cardiovascular disease, and all-cause mortality: a meta-analysis. JAMA. 2011;305(23):2448–2455.

14. Seguin R, Buchner D, Liu J, et al. Sedentary behavior and mortality in older women: the Women's health initiative. Am J Prev Med. 2014;46(2):122–135.

15 Promoting Regular Physical Activity

KEY POINTS

- Physical activity yields multiple health benefits.
- Currently a distinct minority of individuals in the United States are physically active at levels that will yield health benefits.
- Multiple factors impact on the likelihood of maintaining a physically active lifestyle. These include individual factors, community, communication environment (information technology) and physical environment and policy.
- These domains also provide a good mechanism for exploring what is known about effective ways of promoting physical activity.

15.1 INTRODUCTION

The abundant literature on the relationship between regular physical activity and multiple health benefits underscores two concepts. First, physical activity can play multiple positive roles in lowering the risk of chronic disease and improving the daily lives of individuals throughout the lifespan. Second, despite its known benefits the majority of Americans do not participate in enough physical activity. For this reason, this chapter will focus attention on ways that more physical activity can be promoted.

As already indicated in previous chapters in this book, physical activity levels of Americans are typically not enough to obtain the full benefits of an active lifestyle. In 2015, less than half of American adults reported levels of aerobic physical activity consistent with Federal guidelines (1) and 30% of US adults reported high levels of inactivity during leisure time (2). Sadly, in 2015, only 27% of US. high school students reported levels of physical activity that met federal guidelines of 60 minutes or more of physical activity per day (3). For all of these reasons, it is important to explore which ways of promoting physical activity have shown to be successful and which carry the most promise to elevate the levels of physical activity in the future. In addition, as concern has been raised over the level of sedentary behavior, it is important to explore ways of reducing this type of behavior.

15.2 CONCEPTUAL FRAMEWORK FOR FACTORS INFLUENCING PHYSICAL ACTIVITY

The Physical Activity Guidelines for Americans 2018 utilized a framework for conceptualizing factors that impact on physical activity in the United States. This conceptual framework is found in Figure 15.1

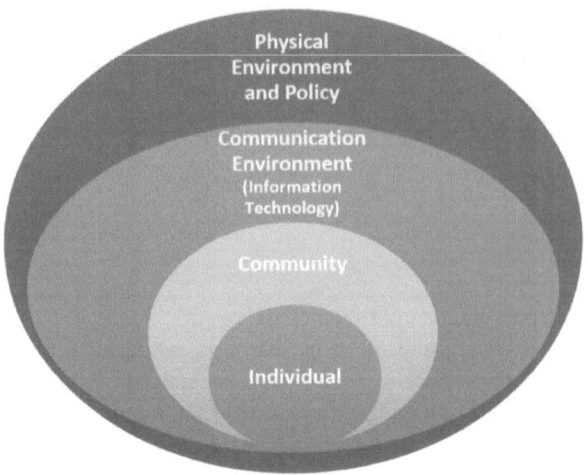

FIGURE 15.1   Social ecological framework.

(From Physical Activity Guidelines Advisory Committee. 2018 Physical Activity Guidelines Advisory Committee. 2018 Physical Activity Committee Scientific Report. Washington, DC US Department of Health and Human Services; 2018.)

As indicated in this figure, there are multiple influences concerning physical activity starting with the individual and then also extending to the community, communication environment as well as the environment in general, and public policy (4). This type of framework has also been used in other areas of behavior such as nutrition where a very similar social ecological model has been employed to help address the factors that need to be addressed when considering more healthful eating in the United Statespopulation.

15.3   INDIVIDUAL LEVEL

The most robust data currently available on effective ways of promoting physical activity comes from initiatives designed to increase physical activity in individuals (5). This is true particularly in the general adult population (6–8), but good data are also available for older adults, postmenopausal women, and youth.

The type of formats used to promote activity in individuals typically involve either one on one sessions or group delivered programs involving structured exercise. Educational approaches have also been employed to teach individuals how to employ various strategies to increase their regular physical activity. Individual interventions for adults typically provide the most flexible ways of tailoring individual advice and support to help individuals meet their needs and preferences. A downside, however, is that they require a higher level of staff involvement and can result in significant costs over the long run. Good examples of this kind of initiative are personal training or various types of structured exercise classes. The same types of interventions have been employed, which target older individuals. These interventions have typically been shown to have a small, but positive effect on physical activity, when compared to no treatment controls.

The PAGA 2018 rated the evidence for individual approaches to promote physical activity as "strong." Oftentimes, these initiatives focus not only on physical activity, but also other health promoting lifestyle activities such as improved diet (more fruit and vegetable consumption) as well as weight loss behaviors. More information on efforts to increase physical activity in older individuals may be found in Chapter 8.

A variety of interventions have been attempted in postnatal individuals, which is a group where adequate physical activity may be difficult to increase or maintain (9). The PAGA 2018 viewed the level of evidence in this area as limited given that there were heterogeneous results in these programs. The most promising of these efforts involve behavior change strategies including goal setting and behavioral self-monitoring. Particularly promising results have occurred in the generally healthy, but inactive women in the postnatal period. (More information concerning these initiatives may be found in Chapter 6).

A variety of individual efforts promoting physical activities in healthy youth have shown considerable promise (10, 11). For this reason, the PAGA 2018 rated this evidence as "strong." The benefits of these programs were enhanced when incorporating family or delivering in school settings. It is particularly important to focus on lifetime physical activities such as leisure time pursuits and noncompetitive sports for all youth. In addition, use of school facilities during nonschool hours as well as improving sidewalk and street design to promote active commuting to and from school appear to be promising strategies. More information on physical activity initiatives in youth maybe found in Chapter 7.

15.4 THEORY-BASED INTERVENTIONS TO INCREASE PHYSICAL ACTIVITY

Most of the interventions involved in lifestyle medicine are based on behavior change. This is, of course, true of efforts to increase physical activity. There are good data now available to suggest that a variety of theory-based interventions carry some efficacy in helping people make behavior changes in their daily lives (12). Multiple studies have looked at various theories of behavior change and the issue of behavior change is becoming more common in medical school curricula. This area is so important that I have devoted a whole section to behavior change theories in the 3rd edition of my *Lifestyle Medicine* textbook (13). Here are some of the behavioral change models that have been showed to be efficacious:

- Health Belief Model (HBM) (14–16)—This model was initially developed in the 1950's and attempts to explain why many individuals were not participating in preventive health services. HBM proposes that the likelihood of individuals would will in a given health behavior largely depends on their perceptions of the following:
  - Severity of Illness(es) or issues
  - Benefits engaging in the behavior
  - Barriers to engaging in the behavior

According to the HBM model individuals are more likely to adopt a health behavior (in this case, more physical activity) if they believe that it is likely to lower their risk of potential illness and also carry benefits from engaging in the action. Many factors prompt those actions such as media campaigns, physician reminders, etc.

Self-efficacy, which has been described as self confidence in a specific behavior, was subsequently added to the HBM model to increase the model's ability to actively predict health behavior. The HBM model has been applied to a variety of long-term health behaviors, including physical activity. While HBM is a highly used model in health behavior research, it has been criticized because some of the constructs such as "cues to action" are difficult to empirically test. In addition, other models have subsequently exhibited stronger predictive ability for health behavior change than HBM. However, the HBM model may be quite useful in the hands of physicians, particularly if they recommend starting a program of increased physical activity.

- Theory of Reasoned Action—Planned Behavior and Integrated Behavior Model—The Theory of Reasoned Action (TRA) stems from premises found in cognitive and social psychology (17, 18). The TRA model proposes that an individual's likelihood of engaging in particular health behavior, such as increased physical activity, can be predicted by the strength of their intention to engage in that behavior. These intentions represent a combination of individuals' attitudes about behavior and the "social norms." The TRA model was extended to what is called the "Theory of Planned Behavior (TPB)." TPB is the concept of perceived facilitators and barriers to behavior. The integrated behavior model (IBM) was a further extension of the TRA and the TPB models. This extension involved adding the importance of evaluating the intention to engage in a behavior (19). All of these models have been demonstrated to be efficacious in various behaviors including increased physical activity.

- Trans Theoretical Model (20, 21)—The Trans Theoretical Model (TTM) is a model of behavior change developed from many different psychological theories. Prochaska and colleagues first described this model by noting that people vary in terms of motivational readiness to make behavioral change, such as quitting smoking. The model is based on people progressing through a series of changes based on "stages of change." This model outlines moving from the pre-contemplation stage to the contemplation stage, followed by the action stage, and finally the maintenance phase. This TTM model been widely adopted throughout behavioral medicine and specifically applied to multiple aspects of behavior, including increased physical activity.

- Social Cognitive Theory (22, 23)—The Social Cognitive Theory (SCT) is a robust behavioral change theory which evolved from Social Learning Theory. It is focused on individuals' response to watching others behavior (also referred to as modeling). Self-efficacy is the main psychological construct for SCT which can be increased through mass experiences, social

modeling, improving physical and emotionally states, and verbal persuasion. This theory has been widely utilized in a variety of different populations and has been specifically applied to increases in physical activity.
- Positive Psychology (24)—Recent interest has emerged in the science of positive psychology and its impact on behavioral change. Positive psychology is defined as the scientific study of "conditions and processes that contribute to the flourishing or optimal functioning of people, groups and institutions." Positive psychology is premised on the belief that the best way to address behavioral changes is leveraging psychological strengths. Positive psychology interventions have been utilized in a variety of chronic diseases such as improvement of well-being and decreases in depression. A typical framework for applying positive psychology includes recommendations to express gratitude to others, recognizing a person's individual strengths and engaging in acts of kindness as well as mindful meditation. All of these considerations may help individuals increase the amount of physical activity in their daily lives.
- Overcoming the Intention/Behavior Gap (25)—Recent attention has been focused on how to overcome the gap between individuals' intentions to actually making the behavior change. Intention alone typically has not been found to be reliable behavior for physical activity changes. To employ the model to increase individuals' actually changing their behavior, physicians should consider issues such as helping the patient plan specific goals and enhance self-efficacy and the positive emotional response.

15.5 COMMUNITY-BASED INTERVENTIONS TO INCREASE PHYSICAL ACTIVITY

A variety of community wide efforts have been undertaken in order to attempt to increase levels of physical activity (26). These community-based approaches have been divided into three domains including: informational, behavioral/social, and policy/environmental approaches.

Community approaches are based on the understanding that many adults report barriers to participation in regular physical activity that relate to community issues. For example, a commonly cited factor is access to facilities or safe places to engage in physical activity. Health-care practitioners can encourage physical activity behavior, but unless individuals have a place in which to be active they are often unable to follow such recommendations. The goal of community-based approaches is to make the community more "physically active friendly" and includes not only general community initiatives, but also specific recommendations for places to promote regular physical activity such as the following:

- *Schools* (27–29)—Many of the physical education and health education curricula are now available to provide a framework for promoting youth physical activity. Many of these strategies have been shown to be effective at increasing physical activity. Unfortunately, there is a paradox in the United States. School buildings and grounds may be the most widely available public resources for physical activity within a community yet are often underutilized. For example, studies of student's engagement in physical activity during leisure time at school suggest that few students use this time to be physically active.

A number of recent studies have shown that factors associated with increased physical activity at schools include the presence of dedicated spaces for physical activity (e.g. sports fields, gyms, access to sports equipment; safe, interesting and newer playgrounds; and sufficient space for physical activity). It is also important to have supervision since this has been shown to increase participation in physical activity.

Unfortunately, many schools have policies in place to restrict access to school grounds by students and community members outside of school hours, thus, leaving these resources underutilized. This is a particular problem in low income communities which often lack other spaces for safe physical activity. A number of community advocacy groups are seeking to find solutions to this issue. In addition, active transport by walking and cycling to and from school can also yield substantial physical activity benefits for children and youth. This was shown by a recent evaluation by Safe Routes to School Program (30). Some states, such as California, have dedicated funding to make physical improvements to environments near schools to enhance safety of individual students who are participating in active transport to and from school.

- *Worksites* (31, 32)—Since many employed adults spend at least half of their waking hours at work, worksites are a natural place to attempt to increase physical activity. Furthermore, physically active jobs have decreased and sedentary jobs have increased over the past few decades. This shift underscores the need to find ways to create a more inviting environment and worksite to increase physical activity.

  A variety of initiatives have shown promise in increasing physical activity in the workplace. These include more flexible work hours and removing potential barriers to physical activity such as establishing facilities and also safe places to store bicycles, and providing showers for employees who wish to engage in physical activity.

  One intriguing initiative was performed by Dishman et al in their "Move to Improve" multisite, randomized, controlled trial. This initiative involved putting together specific plans to combat perceived barriers and improve management support for physical activity. At the end of the 12 week intervention only 2.5% of individuals at control sites engaged in 150 minutes of moderate to vigorous physical activity (MVPA) on a weekly basis, while 51% at the intervention sites met these criteria (33). This suggests that there is great potential in putting together well structured worksite programs and facilities to increase physical activity.

- *Community Organizations*—Numerous community organizations are able to provide facilities and programs with the potential to increase physical activity. These include health clubs, dance studios, swimming pools, sports leagues, etc. Nonprofit organizations such as the YMCA, YWCA, and

Boys & Girls Clubs can also provide places for increased physical activity. In addition, many new private and public housing developments are now including recreational and fitness facilities. Thus, there are many resources throughout the community which can be used to increase physical activity. Unfortunately, however, there are not any well designed, systematic studies about how these facilities and programs within community actually contribute to increased physical levels of individuals in surrounding communities.

• *Public Recreation Facilities and Built Environments*—Public parks and recreation facilities are widely used, with about 80% of the population making some use of municipal facilities. A substantial percentage of individuals also utilize park programs and services (34). Most common activities in a survey of 114 parks in major US cities found that walking and fitness loops were particularly well utilized. Not surprisingly, parks in low income neighborhoods are utilized less and those in high income neighborhoods (34).

It should be noted that parks are also eager to have the public use their facilities as venues for increased physical activity. A survey of 144 recreation center directors in San Diego County showed that 75% were interested in partnering with health professionals to train staff in physical activity leadership (35).

In addition to parks, the design of built environments (e.g., the presence and condition of sidewalks, location and condition green space, availability of public transportation, etc.) has immense potential to impact on participation in physical activity. One survey showed that participants living in the most activity friendly neighborhoods participated in 68–89 more minutes of physical activity per week compared to those living in the least physically activity friendly neighborhoods.

The Community Preventive Sources Task Force now includes recommendations for making built environments more "activity friendly" among its recommendations for increasing physical activity (36). A built environmental strategy combining approved pedestrian land and environmental design to improve pedestrian and bicycle activities can facilitate increased levels of physical activity.

5.5.1 Promoting Use of Place For Physical Activity

A number of health departments have become involved in analyzing ways of attracting more people to utilize such facilities as parks and trails to increase physical activity. These initiatives include publicity campaigns, fun walks with refreshments and tee shirts donated by local businesses, etc. These initiatives have often resulted in recommendations from the public to increase the number of trails available for walking. An example was the "take our trail community program" (36) in the state of Missouri which resulted in a 35% increase in trail use between one month before and one month after a springtime campaign encouraging individuals to utilize trails to obtain more physical activity.

It is important to recognize that often environmental policy interventions designed to increase physical activity need to be justified for cost effectiveness. Such programs as the "CATCH Program" (Coordinated Approach to Child Health) program conducted in Texas showed a large economic benefit with regard to quality of life, year life saved (QALY) (37). This example joins a growing body of literature that shows public initiatives to increase physical activity can generate a high rate of return or investment. A number of programs have now been developed utilizing the Guide for Community Preventive Services which rates the cost effectiveness of various programs.

15.5.2 PRIMARY CARE SETTINGS

A number of different primary care interventions to increase physical activity have been attempted including counseling sessions with primary care providers of short duration (2 to 10 minutes) or long duration (e.g., 40 minutes) (38, 39). Some of these programs provide physician contact only, while others provide a combination of counseling and printed materials.

The evidence cited by the PAGA 2018 report showed that primary care based targeting to improve physical activity was effective when compared to similar "usual care" conditions. The diverse nature of these programs, however, caused the rating to be limited. The primary care setting to encourage physical activity is particularly appealing given that over 70% of adults see their primary care physician at least once a year. Typically, strategies supplemented with counseling and written prescriptions which provide specific activity recommendations are more successful than simply limited amount of counseling (40).

15.5.3 NURSE DELIVERED PROGRAMS

Nurse Delivered Programs have also been shown in a number of studies to have some benefit for increasing physical activities (41, 42). These programs are attractive because Nurse Outreach can be useful given the convenience for population such as frail adults and those with chronic conditions. Nurses also provide personal contact and program customization, which may be particularly useful for behavior change in these populations. The ability of nurses to see patients in their home environment and also involve family members can facilitate physical activity participation. Continuity of care may be an additional benefit from nurse delivered programs.

15.6 COMMUNICATION ENVIRONMENTAL LEVEL

A variety of new information and communication technologies (ICT) have provided additional modalities for increasing the level of physical activity for a wide variety of individuals. These ICTs reach across individuals at every stage in the lifespan. These approaches have been divided into a variety of intervention domains such as wearable activity monitors, telephone, assisted interventions, web-based or internet developed interventions, computer tailored print, mobile phone programs, social media, and interactive video games all of which are designed to promote activity, play or exercise.

- *Wearable Activity Monitors*—The PAGAC 2018 Report rated the evidence that wearable activity monitors such as pedometers, and accelerometers used in conjunction with behavioral strategies can increase levels of physical activity in the general population of adults as well as those with type 2 diabetes as "strong" (43–45). The use of these monitors in conjunction with behavioral strategies expands the possibilities for motivation to increase physical activity. Newer activity monitors have now been shown to have good reliability and fluidity which makes them a promising intervention tool for population wide physical activity promotion.

- *Telephone-assisted Interventions*—A number of interventions have been undertaken over the past few decades involving telephone reminders (46, 47). These interventions have been shown to generate strong evidence to increase physical activity in the general adult population. Since there is a high prevalence of phone ownership these interventions show great promise for increasing physical activity since advice and counseling for adult populations and can be broadly disseminated.

- *Web-based or Internet-delivered Interventions* (46, 48) —A number of new web-based and Internet delivered interventions are now available. The PAGA 2018 rated the effects of these interventions on as "strong" for increasing physical activity in the general adult population. The PAGA 2018 Guidelines also rated the web-based or Internet delivered interventions on individuals with T2DM as "limited" due to the heterogeneity of the studies and results. A particularly attractive aspect of these interventions is the ability to reach a large portion of the population. Thus, even small increases in physical activity in this widely based population could have a significant public health impact.

- *Computer-tailored Print Interventions*—These are interventions that collect information through mailed surveys which are then used to generate computer-tailored mailings containing advice about personalized physical activity and support (49). These interventions seem to have some benefit for the general population when compared to no treatment controls. These interventions may be particularly useful in populations that have lower computer or technology literacy or those living in remote areas where other communication channels are either not present or unreliable.

- *Mobile Phone Programs*—Programs that utilize text messaging appear to have a small to moderate positive effect on physical activity in the general adult population (50–52). There is stronger evidence, however, that smartphone applications increase physical activity in children and adolescents. A positive aspect of the mobile phone platforms is the ability to generate moderate increases in physical activity in some segments of the population. Smartphone applications are applicable particularly in tech savvy children and adolescents and appear to have a stronger association with increases in physical activity in these populations.

- *Social Media*—Physical activity interventions which utilize social media are rapidly developing (53–55). There are fewer long-term trials available, however, for these interventions than for Smartphones. The use of social media with complementary communication channels may increase the likelihood that physical activity messages will yield increases in physical activity in some population groups who are particularly strong users of social media.

- *Interactive Video Games Promoting Active Play or Exercise*—There is some evidence that this type of intervention can increase levels of physical activity (56–58). This is particularly true for youth and those who are active utilizing video games. This approach may also be potentially useful during "in school" times and classroom settings. At the current time, the research in this area is in its infancy.

- *Point of Decision Prompts*—There is good evidence that point of decision prompts such as signage to encourage the use of stairs rather than elevators can have a positive impact on levels of physical activity (59, 60). In addition to signage, messages such as music and art work to increase the likelihood of stair utilization may have some benefit. A clear advantage of this type of intervention is the ubiquitous presence of stairways in most public accommodations.
- *Access to Indoor/Outdoor Facilities*—Having access to either indoor facilities (e.g., gyms, other recreational facilities, health clubs, or swimming pools) and outdoor recreational facilities such as parks, trails, and green spaces is associated with increased levels of physical activity for both children and adults compared to environments that do not have these features (61–63). Since availability and access to these facilities is intertwined with environmental and public policy approaches an overall plan to increase physical activity including access and availability of facilities is very important.

One useful summary of this information can be found at the National Physical Activity Plan (The 2017 US Report Card on Walking and Walkable Communities 2017) (64).

15.7   INTERVENTIONS TO REDUCE SEDENTARY BEHAVIOR

Accumulating evidence has emerged that sedentary behavior can have a significant adverse impact on health consequences. The issue of sedentary behavior is described in more detail in Chapter 14. With this in mind, strategies to promote physical activity should also address ways of reducing sedentary behavior. Data are currently available in three general areas: youth interventions, adult interventions, and worksite interventions.

Moderate data exist that strategies for lowering sedentary behavior in youth such as reduction in television viewing and other screen time behaviors primarily utilized in school based settings have small but consistent results in reducing sedentary behavior (65–67). Given that there are multiple new platforms for media consumption and the associated sedentary times that are associated with these platforms among children, these strategies are important for the future health of our nation. School-based interventions generally focus on reducing screen time amongst children through in class or after school curricula and include messages about ways to reduce screen time. Some evidence has also emerged for home-based interventions although much further research is needed in this area.

With regard to adult interventions, there are some data to suggest that interventions such as education and behavioral approaches to reducing sedentary time may be effective. Combinations of such interventions with programs emphasizing increasing physical activity time, have demonstrated small but consistent impacts on increasing levels of physical activity (68, 69). This is an area where additional research is likely to provide more robust information and tools.

With regard to worksite interventions, those that target workers who perform duties primarily while seated may have significant short-term impacts on reducing sedentary behavior (70, 71). Workplace interventions are appealing because they can be implemented during times when physical activity is generally not feasible. Education and behavioral support are less effective than combining environmental changes as well as education and policy changes designed to reduce prolonged sedentary behavior in the workforce.

15.8 CONCLUSIONS

Lack of physical activity is a significant and pervasive health risk in the United Statesand other industrialized countries. There are multiple interactions between lack of physical activity and adverse health consequences. Despite the abundant knowledge in this area, a distinct minority of Americans are active enough to achieve health benefits. It has been estimated that only 25% of the adult population is active enough to attain benefits outlined by the CDC and the American College of Sports Medicine. Given the low participation rates in physical activity, it is vital to discover ways to promote a more active lifestyle for the population. A number of factors play roles in this area. Perhaps the most coherent framework for this is the social, ecological framework supplied by the Physical Activity Guidelines for Americans Advisory Committee Scientific Report 2018. This model emphasizes the factors that impact on physical activity including individual, community, communication (information technology) and physical environment, and policy (see Figure 15.1).

Similar frameworks have been proposed not only for physical activity but other lifestyle changes for implementing such nutritional guidelines. These frameworks have in common the recognition that multiple factors must be considered to promote behavior change. Such frameworks also emphasize multiple opportunities are available to help people become more physically active by targeting specific factors that impact on physical activity.

CLINICAL APPLICATIONS

- Physicians should routinely recommend increased physical activity in all clinical encounters
- The model proposed by the Physical Activity Guidelines for American Scientific Report 2018 emphasizes the multiple domains where effective promotional strategies maybe employed to increase physical activity. These include: individual, community, communication environment (information technology), physical environment, and policy domains.
- Theory-based behavioral change models exist which can contribute significantly to increasing physical activity physicians should be aware of and utilized the proposed theoretical constructs which have been proven to be effective which are outlined in this chapter.

REFERENCES

1. U.S. Department of Health and Human Services. 2008 Physical Activity Guidelines for Americans. U.S. Department of Health and Human Services (Washington, DC), 2008.
2. U.S. Department of Health and Human Services. Physical activity. Healthy People 2020 Objective Data https://www.healthypeople.gov/2020/topics-objectives/topic/physicalactivity/objectives [Accessed January 13, 2020].

3. Kann L, McManus T, Harris WA, et al. Youth risk behavior surveillance—United States, 2015. MMWR Surveill Summ. 2016;65(SS-6):1–174. doi:10.15585/mmwr.ss6506a1.

4. 2018 Physical Activity Guidelines Advisory Committee. 2018 Physical Activity Guidelines Advisory Committee Scientific Report. U.S. Department of Health and Human Services (Washington, DC), 2018.

5. Centers for Disease Control and Prevention (CDC). Increasing physical activity: a report on recommendations of the task force on Community preventive services. MMWR Recomm Rep. 2001;50(RR-18):1–16.

6. Baxter S, Blank L, Johnson M, et al. Interventions to promote or maintain physical activity during and after the transition to retirement: An evidence synthesis. Public Health Research. NIHR Journals Library (Southampton, UK), 2016.

7. French D, Olander E, Chisholm A, et al. Which behaviour change techniques are most effective at increasing older adults' self-efficacy and physical activity behaviour? A Systematic Review. Ann Behav Med. 2014;48(2):225–234. doi:10.1007/s12160-014-9593-z.

8. Nigg CR, Long CR. A systematic review of single health behavior change interventions vs. Multiple health behavior change interventions among older adults. Transl Behav Med. 2012;2(2):163–179. doi:10.1007/s13142-012-0130-y.

9. Gilinsky AS, Dale H, Robinson C, et al. Efficacy of physical activity interventions in post-natal populations: systematic review, meta-analysis and content coding of behaviour change techniques. Health Psychol Rev. 2015;9(2):244–263. doi:10.1080/17437199.2014.899059.

10. Brown H, Atkin A, Panter J, et al. Family-based interventions to increase physical activity in children: a systematic review, meta-analysis and realist synthesis. Obes Rev. 2016;17(4):345–360. doi:10.1111/obr.12362.

11. Cushing C, Brannon E, Suorsa K, et al. Systematic review and meta-analysis of health promotion interventions for children and adolescents using an ecological framework. J Pediatr Psychol. 2014;39(8):949–962. doi:10.1093/jpepsy/jsu042.

12. Gholami M, Herman C, Ainsworth C, et al. Applying psychological theories to promote lifestyles. In Rippe JM. Lifestyle Medicine (3rd edition). CRC Press (Boca Raton), FL, 2019.

13. Rippe JM. Lifestyle Medicine (3rd edition). CRC Press (Boca Raton, FL), 2019.

14. Becker M, Maiman L. Sociobehavioral determinants of compliance with health care and medical care recommendations. Med Care.1975;13:10–24.

15. Rosenstock I. Why people use health services. The Milbank Memorial Fund Quarterly. 1966;44(3):94–127.

16. Rosenstock I. Historical origins of the health belief model. Health Educ Monogr. 1974;2(4):328–335.

17. Ajzen I, Fishbein M. Understanding Attitudes and Predicting Social Behavior. Prentice-Hall (Englewood Cliffs, NJ), 1980.

18. Fishbein M, Ajzen I. Belief, Attitude, Intention and Behavior: An Introduction to Theory and Research. Addison-Wesley (Reading, MA), 1975.

19. Ajzen I. From intentions to actions: A theory of planned behavior. In J. Kuhl and J. Beckmann: Action-Control: From Cognition to Behavior, 1985, Heidelberg (Springer), pp. 11–39.

20. Bandura A. Principles of Behavior Modification. Holt, Rinehart & Winston (New York), 1969.

21. Skinner, B., Science and Human Behavior. Free Press (New York), 1953.

22. Glanz K, Rimer B, and National Cancer Institute (U.S.), Theory at a Glance: A guide for health promotion practice. NIH Publication no. 97-3896. 1997, Bethesda MD: U.S. Dept. of Health and Human Services, Public Health Service, National Institutes of Health, National Cancer Institute. 48 p.

23. McAlister A, Perry, Parcel G. How individuals, environments, and health behaviors interact: Social cognitive theory. In Glanz K, Rimer B, Viswanath K: Health Behavior and Health Education, pp. 167–188. Jossey-Bass (San Francisco), 2008.

24. Carson S, Cook A, Peabody S et al. The impact of positive psychology on behavioral change and healthy lifestyle choices. In Rippe JM. Lifestyle Medicine (3rd edition). CRC Press (Boca Raton, FL), 2019.

25. Faries M, Kephart W. The intention-behavior gap. In Rippe JM. Lifestyle Medicine (3rd edition). CRC Press (Boca Raton, FL), 2019.

26. Dodson E, Heath G. Policy and environmental supports in promoting physical activity and activing living. In Rippe JM. Lifestyle Medicine (3rd edition). CRC Press (Boca Raton, FL), 2019.

27. Stone E, McKenzie T, Welk G, et al. Effects of physical activity interventions in youth. Review and synthesis. Am J Prev Med. 1998;15(4):298–315.

28. Bangsbo J, Krustrup P, Duda J, et al. The copenhagen consensus Conference 2016: children, youth, and physical activity in schools and during leisure time. Br J Sports Med. 2016;50(19):1177–1178.

29. Hynynen S, van Stralen M, Sniehotta F, et al. A systematic review of school-based interventions targeting physical activity and sedentary behaviour among older adolescents. Int Rev Sport Exerc Psychol. 2016;9(1):22–44.

30. Hoelscher D, Ory M, Dowdy D, et al. Effects of funding allocation for safe routes to school programs on active commuting to school and related behavioral, knowledge, and psychosocial outcomes. Environment and Behavior. 2016;48(1):210–229.

31. Dodson E, Lovegreen S, Elliott M, et al. Worksite policies and environments supporting physical activity in mid-western communities. Am J Health Promot. Sep-Oct 2008;23(1):51–55.

32. United States Department of Labor, Bureau of Labor Statistics. American Time Use Survey Summary, 2014 Results. Available from: https://www.bls.gov/tus/ [Accessed: January 29, 2020].

33. Dishman R, DeJoy D, Wilson M, et al. Move to improve: a randomized workplace trial to increase physical activity. Am J Prev Med. 2009;36(2):133–141.

34. Godbey G, Caldwell L, Floyd M, et al. Contributions of leisure studies and recreation and park management research to the active living agenda. Am J Prev Med. 2005;28(2 Suppl 2):150–158.

35. Moody J, Prochaska J, Sallis J, et al. Viability of parks and recreation centers as sites for youth physical activity promotion. Health Promot Pract. 2004;5(4):438–443.

36. Community Preventive Services Task Force. The Guide to Community Preventive Services: Physical Activity: Built Environment Approaches Combining Transportation System Interventions with Land Use and Environmental Design. 2016. Available from: http://thecommunityguide.org/taskforce [Accessed: January 15, 2020].

37. Brown H, Perez A, Li Y, et al. The cost-effectiveness of a school-based overweight program. Int J Behav Nutr Phys Act. 2007;4:47.

38. Orrow G, Kinmonth A, Sanderson S, et al. Republished research: effectiveness of physical activity promotion based in primary care: systematic review and meta-analysis of randomised controlled trials. Br J Sports Med. 2013;47(1):27. doi:10.1136/bjsports-2012-e1389rep.

39. Arsenijevic J, Groot W. Physical activity on prescription schemes (PARS): Do programme characteristics influence effectiveness? Results of a systematic review and meta-analyses. BMJ Open. 2017;7(2):1–14.e012156. doi:10.1136/bmjopen-2016- 012156.

40. Denison E, Vist G, Underland V, et al. Interventions aimed at increasing the level of physical activity by including organised follow-up: a systematic review of effect. BMC Fam Prac. 2014;15(1):2–24. doi:10.1186/1471-2296-15-120.

41. Richards EA, Cai Y. Integrative review of nurse-delivered community-based physical activity promotion. Appl Nurs Res. 2016;31:132–138. doi:10.1016/j.apnr.2016.02.004.

42. Holland S, Greenberg J, Tidwell L, et al. Community-based health coaching, exercise, and health service utilization. J Aging Health. 2005;17(6):697–716. doi:10.1177/0898264305277959.

43. Funk M, Taylor E. Pedometer-based walking interventions for free-living adults with type 2 diabetes: a systematic review. Curr Diabetes Rev. 2013;9(6):462–471. doi:10.217 4/15733998113096660084.

44. Goode A, Hall K, Batch B, et al. The impact of interventions that integrate accelerometers on physical activity and weight loss: a systematic review. Ann Behav Med. 2017;51(1):79–93. doi:10.1007/s12160-016-9829-1.

45. Mansi S, Milosavljevic S, Baxter GD, et al. A systematic review of studies using pedometers as an intervention for musculoskeletal diseases. BMC Musculoskelet Disord. 2014;(2):231. doi:10.1186/1471-2474-15-231.

46. Foster C, Richards J, Thorogood M, et al. Remote and web 2.0 interventions for promoting physical activity. Cochrane Database Syst Rev. 2013;(9). doi:10.1002/14651858. CD010395.pub2.

47. Goode AD, Reeves MM, Eakin EG. Telephone-delivered interventions for physical activity and dietary behavior change: an updated systematic review. Am J Prev Med. 2012;42(1):81–88. doi:10.1016/j.amepre.2011.08.025.

48. Davies C, Spence J, Vandelanotte C, et al. Meta-analysis of internet delivered interventions to increase physical activity levels. Int J Behav Nutr Phys Act. 2012;9:52. doi:10.1186/1479-5868-9-52.

49. Short C, James E, Plotnikoff R, et al. Efficacy of tailored-print interventions to promote physical activity: a systematic review of randomised trials. Int J Behav Nutr Phys Act. 2011;8:113. doi:10.1186/1479-5868-8-113.

50. Buchholz S, Wilbur J, Ingram D, et al. Physical activity text messaging interventions in adults: a systematic review. Worldviews Evid Based Nurs. 2013;10(3):163–173. doi:10.1111/wvn.12002.

51. Bort-Roig J, Gilson N, Puig-Ribera A, et al. Measuring and influencing physical activity with smartphone technology: a systematic review. Sports Med. 2014;44(5):671–686. doi:10.1007/s40279-014-0142-5.

52. Pfaeffli Dale L, Dobson R, Whittaker R, et al. The effectiveness of mobile-health behaviour change interventions for cardiovascular disease self-management: a systematic review. Eur J Prev Cardiol. 2016;23(8):801–817. doi:10.1177/2047487315613462.

53. Maher C, Lewis L, Ferrar K, et al. Are health behavior change interventions that use online social networks effective? A systematic review. J Med Internet Res. 2014;16(2):e40.

54. Mita G, Ni Mhurchu C, Jull A. Effectiveness of social media in reducing risk factors for non-communicable diseases: a systematic review and meta-analysis of randomized controlled trials. Nutr Rev. 2016;74(4):237–247. doi:10.1093/nutrit/nuv106.

55. Williams G, Hamm M, Shulhan J, et al. Social media interventions for diet and exercise behaviours: a systematic review and meta-analysis of randomised controlled trials. BMJ Open. 2014;4(2):e003926.

56. Norris E, Hamer M, Stamatakis E. Active video games in schools and effects on physical activity and health: a systematic review. J Pediatr. 2016;172:40–46.e5. doi:10.1016/j. jpeds.2016.02.001.

57. Valenzuela T, Okubo Y, Woodbury A, et al. Adherence to technology-based exercise programs in older adults: a systematic review. J Geriatr Phys Ther. 2016.

58. Liang Y, Lau P. Effects of active videogames on physical activity and related outcomes among healthy children: a systematic review. Games Health J. 2014;3(3):122–144. doi:10.1089/g4h.2013.0070.

59. Jennings C, Yun L, Loitz C, et al. A systematic review of interventions to increase stair use. Am J Prev Med. 2017;52(1):106–114. doi:10.1016/j.amepre.2016.08.014.

60. Eves F, Webb O, Mutrie N. A workplace intervention to promote stair climbing: Greater effects in the overweight. Obesity (Silver Spring). 2006;14(12):2210–2216.

61. Calogiuri G, Chroni S. The impact of the natural environment on the promotion of active living: an integrative systematic review. BMC Public Health. 2014;14:873. doi:10.1186/1471-2458-14-873.

62. Hunter R, Christian H, Veitch J, et al. The impact of interventions to promote physical activity in urban green space: a systematic review and recommendations for future research. Soc Sci Med. 2015;124:246–256. doi:10.1016/j.socscimed.2014.11.051.

63. Bancroft C, Joshi S, Rundle A, et al. Association of proximity and density of parks and objectively measured physical activity in the United States: a systematic review. Soc Sci Med. 2015;138:22–30. doi:10.1016/j.socscimed.2015.05.034.

64. National Physical Activity Plan. The 2017 United States Report Card on Walking and Walkable Communities. http://physicalactivityplan.org/projects/walking-rc.html [Accessed February 10, 2020].

65. van Grieken A, Ezendam N, Paulis W, et al. Primary prevention of overweight in children and adolescents: a meta-analysis of the effectiveness of interventions aiming to decrease sedentary behaviour. Int J Behav Nutr Phys Act. 2012;9(2):61. doi:10.1186/1479-5868-9-61.

66. Wahi G, Parkin PC, Beyene J, et al. Effectiveness of interventions aimed at reducing screen time in children: a systematic review and meta-analysis of randomized controlled trials. Arch Pediatr Adolesc Med. 2011;165(11):979–986. doi:10.1001/archpediatrics.2011.122.

67. Biddle S, O'Connell S, Braithwaite R. Sedentary behaviour interventions in young people: a meta-analysis. Br J Sports Med. 2011;45(11):937–942. 10.1136/bjsports-2011-090205.

68. Prince S, Saunders T, Gresty K, et al. A comparison of the effectiveness of physical activity and sedentary behaviour interventions in reducing sedentary time in adults: a systematic review and meta-analysis of controlled trials. Obes Rev. 2014;15(11):905–919. doi:10.1111/obr.12215.

69. Martin A, Fitzsimons C, Jepson R, et al. EuroFIT consortium. Interventions with potential to reduce sedentary time in adults: systematic review and meta-analysis. Br J Sports Med. 2015;49(16):1056–1063. doi:10.1136/bjsports-2014-094524.

70. Chu A, Ng S, Tan C, et al. A systematic review and meta-analysis of workplace intervention strategies to reduce sedentary time in white-collar workers. Obes Rev. 2016; 17(5):467–481. doi:10.1111/obr.12388.

71. Shrestha N, Ijaz S, Kukkonen-Harjula KT, et al. Workplace interventions for reducing sitting at work. Cochrane Database Syst Rev. 2015;1:Cd010912. doi:10.1002/14651858. CD010912.pub2.

Appendix A

2018 PAR-Q+

The Physical Activity Readiness Questionnaire for Everyone

The health benefits of regular physical activity are clear; more people should engage in physical activity every day of the week. Participating in physical activity is very safe for MOST people. This questionnaire will tell you whether it is necessary for you to seek further advice from your doctor OR a qualified exercise professional before becoming more physically active.

GENERAL HEALTH QUESTIONS

Please read the 7 questions below carefully and answer each one honestly: check YES or No	YES	NO
1) Has your doctor ever said that you have a heart condition☐OR high blood pressure☐?	☐	☐
2) Do you feel pain in your chest at rest, during your daily activities of living, **OR** when you do physical activity	☐	☐
3) Do you lose balance because of dizziness **OR** have you lost consciousness in the last 12 months? (Please answer NO if your dizziness was associated with over-breathing (including during vigorous exercise).	☐	☐
4) Have you ever been diagnosed with another chronic medical condition (other than heart disease or high blood pressure)? PLEASE LIST CONDITION(S) HERE:_____	☐	☐
5) Are you currently taking prescribed medications for a chronic medical condition: PLEASE LIST CONDITION(S) AND MEDICATIONS HERE:_____	☐	☐
6) Do you currently have (or have had within the past 12 months) a bone, joint, or soft tissue (muscle, ligament, or tendon) problem that could be made worse by becoming more physically active? (Please answer NO if you had a problem in the past, but it does not limit your current ability to be physically active). PLEASE LIST CONDITION(S) HERE:_____	☐	☐
7) Has your doctor ever said that you should only do medically supervised physical activity?	☐	☐

☑ **If you answered NO to all of the questions above, you are cleared for physical activity. Go to page 4 to sign the PARTICIPANT DECLARATION. You do not need to complete Pages 2 and 3.**

➢ Start becoming much more physically active – start slowly and build up gradually.
➢ Follow International Physical Activity Guidelines for your age (www.who.int/dietphysicalactivity/en/).
➢ You may take part in a health and fitness appraisal.
➢ If you are over the age of 45 and **NOT** accustomed to regular vigorous to maximal effort exercise, consult a qualified exercise professional before engaging in this intensity of exercise.
➢ If you have any further questions, contact a qualified exercise professional.

○ **If you answered YES to one or more of the questions above, COMPLETE PAGES 2 AND 3.**

⚠ **Delay becoming more active if:**
✓ You have a temporary illness such as a cold or fever, it is best to wait until you feel better.
✓ You are pregnant – talk to your health care practitioner, your physician, a qualified exercise professional, and/or complete the ePARmed-X+ at www.eparmedx.com before becoming more physically active.
✓ Your health changes – answer the questions of Pages 2and 3 of this document and/or talk to your doctor or a qualified exercise professional before continuing with any physical activity program.

2018 PAR-Q+

FOLLOW-UP QUESTIONS ABOUT YOUR MEDICAL CONDITION(S)

1. Do you have Arthritis, Osteoporosis, or Back Problems?
If the above condition(s) is/are present answer questions 1a-1c   If NO☐ go to question 2

1a Do you have difficulty controlling your condition with medications or other physician prescribed therapies?
(Answer NO if you are not currently taking medications or other treatments)   YES ☐   NO ☐

1b Do you have joint problems causing pain, a recent fracture or fracture caused by osteoporosis or cancer, displaced vertebra (e.g., spondylolisthesis), and/or spondylolysis/pars defect (a crack in the bony ring on the back of the spinal column)?   YES ☐   NO ☐

1c Have you had steroid injections or taken steroid tablets regularly for more than 3 months?   YES ☐   NO ☐

2. Do you have Cancer of any kind?
If the above condition(s) is/are present, answer questions 2a-2b   If NO☐ go to question 3

2a Does your cancer diagnosis include any of the following types; lung/bronchogenic, multiple myeloma (cancer of plasma cells), head, and neck?   YES ☐   NO ☐

2b Are you currently receiving cancer therapy (such as chemotherapy or radiotherapy)?   YES ☐   NO ☐

3. Do you have a Heart or Cardiovascular Condition? *This includes Coronary Artery Disease, Heart Failure, Diagnosed Abnormality of Heart Rhythm*
If the above condition(s) is/are present, answer questions 3a-3d   If NO☐ go to question 4

3a Do you have difficulty controlling your condition with medications or other physician-prescribed therapies? (Answer NO if you are not currently taking medications or other treatments)   YES ☐   NO ☐

3b Do you have an irregular heart beat that required medical management?
(e.g., atrial fibrillation, premature ventricular contraction)   YES ☐   NO ☐

3c Do you have chronic heart failure?   YES ☐   NO ☐

3d Do you have diagnosed coronary artery (cardiovascular) disease and have not participated in regular physical activity in the last 2 months?   YES ☐   NO ☐

4. Do you have High Blood Pressure?
If the above condition(s) is/are present, answer questions 4a-4b   If NO☐ go to question 5

4a Do you have difficulty controlling your condition with medications or other physician-prescribed therapies? (Answer NO if you are not currently taking medications or other treatments)   YES ☐   NO ☐

4b Do you have a resting blood pressure equal to or greater than 160/90 mmHg with or without medication? (Answer YES if you do not know your resting blood pressure)   YES ☐   NO ☐

5. Do you have any Metabolic Conditions? *This Includes Type 1 Diabetes, Type 2 Diabetes, Pre-Diabetes*
If the above condition(s) is/are present, answer questions 5a-5e   If NO☐ go to question 6

5a Do you often have difficulty controlling your blood sugar levels with foods, medications, or other physician-prescribed therapies?   YES ☐   NO ☐

5b Do you often suffer from signs and symptoms of low blood sugar (hypoglycemia) following exercise and/or during activities of daily living? Signs of hypoglycemia may include shakiness, nervousness, unusual irritability, abnormal sweating, dizziness or light-headedness, mental confusion, difficulty speaking, weakness, or sleepiness.   YES ☐   NO ☐

5c Do you have any signs or symptoms of diabetes complications such as heart or vascular disease and/or complications affecting your eyes, kidneys, **OR** the sensation in your toes and feet?   YES ☐   NO ☐

5d. Do you have other metabolic conditions (such as current pregnancy-related diabetes, chronic kidney disease or liver problems)?   YES ☐   NO ☐

5e Are you planning to engage in what for you is unusually high (or vigorous) intensity exercise in the near future?   YES ☐   NO ☐

2018 PAR-Q+

6. **Do you have any Mental Health Problems or Learning Difficulties?** *This includes Alzheimer's Dementia, Depression, Anxiety Disorder, Eating Disorder, Psychotic Disorder, Intellectual Disability, Down Syndrome*
If the above condition(s) is/are present, answer questions 6a-6b   If **NO** go to question 7

6a Do you have difficulty controlling your condition with medications or other physician-prescribed therapies? (Answer **NO** if you are not currently taking medications or other treatments)   YES ☐ NO ☐

6b Do you ALSO have back problems affecting nerves or muscles?   YES ☐ NO ☐

7. **Do you have a Respiratory Disease?** *This includes Chronic Obstructive Pulmonary Disease, Asthma, Pulmonary High Blood Pressure*
If the above condition(s) is/are present, answer questions 7a-7d   If **NO** go to question 8

7a Do you have difficulty controlling your condition with medications or other physician-prescribed therapies? (Answer **NO** if you are not currently taking medications or other treatments)   YES ☐ NO ☐

7b Has your doctor ever said your blood oxygen level is low at rest or during exercise and/or that you require supplemental oxygen therapy?   YES ☐ NO ☐

7c If asthmatic, do you currently have symptoms of chest tightness, wheezing, labored breathing, consistent cough (more than 2 days/week), or have you used your rescue medication more than twice in the last week?   YES ☐ NO ☐

7d Has your doctor ever said you have high blood pressure in the blood vessels of your lungs?   YES ☐ NO ☐

8. Do you have a Spinal Cord Injury? *This includes Tetraplegia and Paraplegia*
If the above condition(s) is/are present, answer questions 8a-8c   If **NO** go to question 9

8a Do you have difficulty controlling your condition with medications or other physician-prescribed therapies?
(Answer **NO** if you are not currently taking medications or other treatments)   YES ☐ NO ☐

8b Do you commonly exhibit low resting blood pressure significant enough to cause dizziness, light-headedness, and/or fainting?   YES ☐ NO ☐

8c Has your physician indicated that you exhibit sudden bouts of high blood pressure (known as Autonomic Dysreflexia)   YES ☐ NO ☐

9. **Have you had a Stroke?** *This includes Transient Ischemic Attack (TIA) or Cerebrovascular Event*
If the above condition(s) is/are present, answer questions 9a-9c   If **NO** go to question 10

9a Do you have difficulty controlling you condition with medications or other physician-prescribed therapies?
(Answer **NO** if you are not currently taking medications or other treatments)   YES ☐ NO ☐

9b Do you have any impairment in walking or mobility?   YES ☐ NO ☐

9c Have you experienced a stroke or impairment in nerves or muscles in the past 6 months?   YES ☐ NO ☐

10. **Do you have any other medical condition not listed above or do you have two or more medical conditions?**
If you have other medical conditions, answer questions 10a-10c   If **NO** read the Page 4 recommendations

10a Have you experienced a blackout, fainted, or lost consciousness as a result of a head injury within the last 12 months **OR** have you had a diagnosed concussion within the last 12 months?   YES ☐ NO ☐

10b Do you have a medical condition that is not listed (such as epilepsy, neurological conditions, kidney problems)?   YES ☐ NO ☐

10c Do you currently live with two or more medical conditions?   YES ☐ NO ☐
PLEASE LIST YOUR MEDICAL CONDITIONS(S)_____
AND ANY RELATED MEDICATIONS HERE:_____

> GO to Page 4 for recommendations about your current
> medical condition(s) and sign the PARTICIPANT DECLARATION.

2018 PAR-Q+

☑ **If you answered NO to all of the follow-up questions about your medical condition, you are ready to become more physically active – sign the PARTICIPANT DECLARATION below:**
> It is advised that you consult a qualified exercise professional to help you develop a safe and effective physical activity plan to meet your health needs.
> You are encouraged to start slowly and build up gradually – 20 to 60 minutes of low to moderate intensity exercise, 3-5 days per week including aerobic and muscle strengthening exercises.
> As you progress, you should aim to accumulate 150 minutes or more of moderate intensity physical activity per week.
> If you are over the age of 45 yr and **NOT** accustomed to regular vigorous to maximal effort exercise, consult a qualified exercise professional before engaging in this intensity of exercise.

● If you answered **YES** to **one or more of the follow-up questions** about your medical condition:
You should seek further information before becoming more physically active or engaging in a fitness appraisal. You should complete the specially designed online screening and exercise recommendations program – the ePARmed-X+at www.eparmedx.com and/or visit a qualified exercise professional to work through the ePARmed-X+ and for further information.

⚠ Delay becoming more active if:
✓ You have a temporary illness such as a cold or fever; it is best to wait until you feel better.
✓ You are pregnant – talk to your health care practioner, you physician, and qualified exercise professional, and/or complete the ePARmed-X+ at www.eparmedx.com before becoming more physically active.
✓ Your health changes – talk to your doctor or qualified exercise professional before continuing with any physical activity program.

• You are encouraged to photocopy the PAR-Q+. You must use the entire questionnaire and NO changes are permitted.
• The authors, the PAR-Q+ Collaboration, partner organizations, and their agents assume no liability for persons who undertake physical activity and/or make use of the PAR-Q+ or ePARmed-X+. If in doubt after completing the questionnaire, consult your doctor prior to physical activity.

NAME _____ DATE _____

Reprinted with permission from the PAR-Q+ Collaboration and the authors of the PAR-**Q**+ (Dr. Darren Warburton, Dr. Norman Gledhill, Dr. Veronica Jamnik, and Dr. Shannon Bredin)

Appendix B

RLI FITNESS WALKING PROGRAMS

BLUE PROGRAM*

Week	1–2	3–4	5	6	7–8	9	10	11	12–13	14	15–16	17–18	19–20
WARM-UP (mins. before walk stretches)	5–7	5–7	5–7	5–7	5–7	5–7	5–7	5–7	5–7	5–7	5–7	5–7	5–7
MILEAGE	1.0	1.25	1.5	1.5	1.75	2.0	2.0	2.0	2.25	2.5	2.5	2.75	3.0
STEPS	2,000	2,500	3,000	3,000	3,250	4,000	4,000	4,000	4,500	5,000	5,000	5,500	6,000
PACE (mph)	3.0	3.0	3.0	3.5	3.5	3.5	3.75	3.75	3.75	3.75	4.0	4.0	4.0
HEART RATE (% of max)	60	60	60	60–70	60–70	60–70	60–70	70	70	70	70	70–80	70–80
COOLDOWN (mins. after walk stretches)	5–7	5–7	5–7	5–7	5–7	5–7	5–7	5–7	5–7	5–7	5–7	5–7	5–7
FREQUENCY (times per week)	5	5	5	5	5	5	5	5	5	5	5	5	5

* At the end of the 20-week fitness protocol, retest yourself to establish your new program.

GREEN PROGRAM*

Week	1–2	3–4	5–6	7	8–9	10–12	13	14	15–16	17–18	19–20
WARM-UP (mins. before walk stretches)	5–7	5–7	5–7	5–7	5–7	5–7	5–7	5–7	5–7	5–7	5–7
MILEAGE	1.5	1.75	2.0	2.0	2.25	2.5	2.75	2.75	3.0	3.25	3.5
STEPS	3,000	3,500	4,000	4,000	4,500	5,000	5,500	5,500	6,000	6,500	6,500
PACE (mph)	3.0	3.0	3.0	3.5	3.5	3.5	3.5	4.0	4.0	4.0	4.0
HEART RATE (% of max)	60–70	60–70	60–70	70	70	70	70	70–80	70–80	70–80	70–80
COOLDOWN (mins. after walk stretches)	5–7	5–7	5–7	5–7	5–7	5–7	5–7	5–7	5–7	5–7	5–7
FREQUENCY (times per week)	5	5	5	5	5	5	5	5	5	5	5

* At the end of the 20-week fitness protocol, retest yourself to establish your new program.

YELLOW PROGRAM*

Week	1	2	3–4	5	6–8	9–10	11–12	13–14	15	16–17	18–20
WARM-UP (mins. before walk stretches)	5–7	5–7	5–7	5–7	5–7	5–7	5–7	5–7	5–7	5–7	5–7
MILEAGE	2.0	2.25	2.5	2.75	2.75	3.0	3.0	3.25	3.5	3.5	4.0
STEPS	4,000	4,500	5,000	5,500	5,500	6,000	6,000	6,500	7,000	7,000	8,000
PACE (mph)	3.0	3.0	3.0	3.0	3.5	3.5	4.0	4.0	4.0	4.5	4.5
HEART RATE (% of max)	70	70	70	70	70	70	70–80	70–80	70–80	70–80	70–80
COOLDOWN (mins. after walk stretches)	5–7	5–7	5–7	5–7	5–7	5–7	5–7	5–7	5–7	5–7	5–7
FREQUENCY (times per week)	5	5	5	5	5	5	5	5	5	5	5

* At the end of the 20-week fitness protocol, you may either retest yourself and move to a new fitness-walking category or follow the Yellow Maintenance Program for a lifetime of fitness walking.

ORANGE PROGRAM*

Week	1	2	3–4	5	6	7	8	9–10	11–14	15–20
WARM-UP (mins. before walk stretches)	5–7	5–7	5–7	5–7	5–7	5–7	5–7	5–7	5–7	5–7
MILEAGE	2.5	2.75	3.0	3.25	3.25	3.5	3.75	4.0	4.0	4.0
STEPS	5,000	5,500	6,000	6,500	6,500	7,000	7,500	8,000	8,000	8,000
PACE (mph)	3.5	3.5	3.5	3.5	4.0	4.0	4.0	4.0	4.5	4.5
INCLINE/WEIGHT **										
HEART RATE (% of max)	50–70	50–70	50–70	50–70	50–70	50–70	50–70	50–70	50–70	
COOLDOWN (mins. after walk stretches)	5–7	5–7	5–7	5–7	5–7	5–7	5–7	5–7	5–7	5–7
FREQUENCY (times per week)	5	5	5	5	5	5	5	5	5	3

* At the end of the 20-week fitness protocol, follow the Orange/Red Maintenance Program for a lifetime of fitness walking.

** During weeks 15–20, arm weights or incline may be added to increase intensity.

RED PROGRAM*

Week	1	2	3	4	5	6	7–20
WARM-UP (mins. before walk stretches)	5–7	5–7	5–7	5–7	5–7	5–7	5–7
MILEAGE	3.0	3.25	3.5	3.5	3.75	4.0	4.0
STEPS	6,000	6,500	7,000	7,000	7,500	8,000	8,000
PACE (mph)	4.0	4.0	4.0	4.5	4.5	4.5	4.5
INCLINE/WEIGHT **							
HEART RATE (% of max)	70	70	70	70–80	70–80	70–80	70–80
COOLDOWN (mins. after walk stretches)	5–7	5–7	5–7	5–7	5–7	5–7	5–7
FREQUENCY (times per week)	5	5	5	5	5	5	3

* At the end of the 20-week fitness protocol, follow the Orange/Red Maintenance Program for a lifetime of fitness walking.

** During weeks 15–20, arm weights or incline may be added to increase intensity.

YELLOW MAINTENANCE PROGRAM

WARM-UP	5–7 minutes before walk stretches
AEROBIC WORK OUT	mileage: 4.0; pace: 4.5 mph
HEART RATE	70–80% of maximum
COOLDOWN	5–7 minutes after walk stretches
FREQUENCY	3–5 times per week
WEEKLY MILEAGE	12–20 minutes
WEEKLY STEPS	24,000–40,000

ORANGE/RED MAINTENANCE PROGRAM

WARM-UP	5–7 minutes before walk stretches
AEROBIC WORK OUT	mileage: 4.0; pace: 4.5 mph
	weight/incline: Add weights to upper body or add hill walking as needed to keep heart rate in target zone (70–80% of predicted maximum)
HEART RATE	70–80% of maximum
COOLDOWN	5–7 minutes after walk stretches
FREQUENCY	3–5 times per week
WEEKLY MILEAGE	12–20 minutes
WEEKLY STEPS	24,000–40,000

Source: Rippe JM, Ward A: The Rockport Walking Program, Prentice Hall Press (New York), 1989.

Appendix C

AT-HOME STRENGTH TRAINING PROGRAM

Half curl-up. Lie on your back, knees bent, feet close to the buttocks. Cross your arms over your chest. Slowly curl your body forward, lifting your head, neck, shoulders, and upper back off the floor. Your lower back should remain flat, in contact with the floor. Then, in a smooth, slow motion, lower your body back down to the floor. One curl should take four seconds (two to curl up, two to lower). For the stomach and upper back.

Alternating knee touch. Lie on your back, hands behind head, fingers interlocked, elbows out. Now bend your knees and lift them so the lower portion of both legs are resting on a chair or bench. Keeping your lower back on the floor, slowly curl your upper body forward and rotate your trunk so your right elbow touches the left knee and vice versa. If you can't quite reach your knee with your elbow, move your knee in slightly so your elbow can reach it, allowing you to complete the exercise. For the waist and the stomach.

Double flutter. Lie on your stomach, hands resting comfortably under your chin, legs straight and together. Tighten your buttocks and slowly lift both feet two to six inches off the ground, then lower your feet slowly. For buttocks and thighs.

Chest raise. Lie on your stomach, hands behind head, fingers interlocked. Keeping your feet on the ground, slowly lift your head and upper body up from the floor. Hold for two seconds, and return to the ground slowly. If you can't do this alone, ask a partner to hold your feet down. For the lower back, buttocks, and hamstrings.

Push-ups. Do the same push-ups you did for the push-up test earlier in this section. For the arms, shoulders, and chest.

Inverted push-ups. Sit with your legs stretched out in front of you. Your palms are flat on the floor behind you, your arms are placed shoulder-width apart. Now raise yourself until your elbows are nearly straight but not locked, your legs are outstretched, and your toes are pointed. Lower yourself until your buttocks just touch the floor, and repeat. For the arms, shoulders, and upper back.

Lunges. Begin in a standing position, hands on hips. Step forward with the right foot, bending on one knee and dipping, with your left leg outstretched behind you. Step back to the starting position. Step forward with the right foot, repeating dipping and outstretching motions. For the thighs (quads and hamstrings).

Three-way leg lift. Stand near a wall or piece of furniture for support. While standing on your left leg with the knee straight but not locked, slowly raise the right leg, with the toe pointed, straight up in front of you, six to twelve inches. Hold for two seconds.

Again in a smooth motion, return to the beginning position and slowly extend the leg out behind you, lifting six to twelve inches off the ground, toes pointed. Hold for two seconds. Return your leg to the beginning position.

Repeat with the left leg. You should gradually build to do this exercise without resting between position changes. For added resistance, use light ankle weights. For hips, buttocks, and thighs (gluteus, quads, and hamstrings).

Heel lifts. Stand on one step, balancing on the balls of your feet, near a wall or railing. Slowly rise up onto your toes, hold for two seconds, then return to a balanced position. Now let your heels drop off the step, hold for one second, and return to a balanced position. This can also be done one foot at a time, or with ankle weights. For calves, ankles, and feet.

Classic curl. Stand with legs about shoulder width apart. Grasp a dumbbell with each hand, arms extended at the side, palms facing in. Bending at the elbows, curl the weight in toward your body, up to about shoulder height. Your palms should be facing you as you lift the weights. You can do both arms at the same time, or alternate. Remember to breathe smoothly as you lift. For front of the arms (biceps).

Triceps teaser. Standing with legs about shoulder-width apart, grasp the end of one dumbbell with both hands and place your arms above your head. Your elbows should be bent, your hands grasping the weight behind your head. Slowly extend both arms over your head, hold for two seconds, and return to the starting position. For back of the arms.

From Exercise Exchange Program. Simon & Schuster, N.Y. 1992. Used with permission of author.

Index

Pages in *italics* and **bold** refer to figures and tables respectively.

36 item Short-Form Survey (SF-36), *see* Short Form Health Survey (SF-36)

A

Absolute *vs.* relative intensity, 19–20
Academic achievement, youth, 83
Access to indoor/outdoor facilities, 182
Adiposity, 81–82
Adiposity-based chronic disease (ABCD), 58
Adults, 33–34, **36**
　interventions, 182–183
Aerobic Center Longitudinal Research Study, 112
Aerobic physical activity, 6, 18, 20–21, 59, 67, *104*, 112, 113–114, 155–157
Affect, defined, 126
African Americans, 34
Age related memory impairment (ARMI), 92
All-cause mortality, 3, 5, 68, 165–168, *166*, *167*
Alzheimer disease (AD), 8, 72, 92, 107, 124–125
Alzheimer's Disease Foundation, 130
American Academy of Family Practice, 17
American Academy of Geriatrics, 141
American Academy of Orthopedic Surgeons, 141
American Academy of Pediatrics, 141
American Association of Retired Persons (AARP), 68, 71
American Cancer Society, 49, 50, 68, 70
American College of Cardiology (ACC), 30, 103, 141
American College of Lifestyle Medicine (ACLM), 2, 17, 141, 142
American College of Preventive Medicine, 17, 141
American College of Sports Medicine (ACSM), 2, 7, 22, 24, 49, 61, 67, 75, 80, 112, 141, 142, 154, 155
American College of Sports Medicine Complete Guide to Fitness and Health (Bushman), 159
American Diabetes Association (ADA), 2, 6–7, 57, 59, 61
American Endocrinology Society, 58
American Heart Association (AHA), 2, 7, 11, 17, 25, 30, 37, 67, 80, 103, 123, 129–130, 141
American Institute for Cancer Research (AICR), 49, 70
American Journal of Lifestyle Medicine, 17
American Medical Association, 141

American Stroke Association (ASA), 8, 25, 35, 123, 129–130
Anaerobic physical activities, 18
Anxiety, 3, 8, 126–127; *see also* Depression

B

Balance, 18, 159
Balke protocol, 143
Bariatric surgery, 114
Benson, H., 160
Biomarkers of brain health, 125
Bladder cancer, 48
Blood glucose, 79
Blood lipids, 36–37
Blood pressure
　categories of, **36**
　control of, 30, 141
　diastolic, 36, **36**, 104
　guidelines for, 35
　high, 6, 35, 83, 130
　level, *104*
　management, 142
　response, *104*
　systolic, 35, **36**, 104, 116
　treatment of, 9
　untreated, 25
Body composition, 74
Body mass index (BMI), 39, 50, 144
Body position, 19
Body weight, 81–82
Bone health, 73, 82
Bone mineral density (BMD), 73
Bone strengthening activities, 18
Brain cancer, 49
Brain derived neurotrophic factor (BDNF), 93
Brain health, 8, 35, 72; *see also* Optimal brain health; Osteoporosis
　affect, 126
　anxiety, 126–127
　biomarkers of, 125
　cognitive function, 124–125
　cognitive reserve, 128–129
　defined, 123
　depression, 127
　overview, 123
　quality of life (QoL), 125–126
　sleep, 127–128
Breast cancer, 48, 70
Breast health, 71–72

Bruce protocol, 143
Burnout, 148
Bushman, B., 159

C

Canadian Diabetes Canada, 59
Cancer(s), 45–54
    bladder, 48
    brain, 49
    breast, 48, 70
    clinical recommendations, **51**
    colon, 48, 71
    endometrial, 48, 71
    esophageal, 48
    gastric, 48
    head and neck, 48
    health-enhancing physical activity, 49–50
    hematologic, 48
    lung, 48, 71
    as a metabolic disease, 52–53
    mortality, 169
    ovarian, 49, 71
    overview, 45–46
    pancreatic, 49
    prostate, 49, 103
    protective effects, 48–49
    rectal, 49
    renal, 48
    risk of, 3
    sedentary behavior and, 50
    thyroid, 49
    types/variety of, 9, 17
    women's health, 70–71
Cancer Prevention Study II (CPS-II), 68
Cancer survivor, 101–103
Cardiovascular disease (CVD), 29–40, 94, *105*,
        138; *see also* Diabetes; Diseases;
        Obesity; Overweight
    atherosclerotic, 80
    brain health, 35
    chronic diseases, 3–6
    diabetes, 38
    effects on risk factors for, 116–117
    heart disease, 39–40
    heart failure (HF), 38
    hypertension, 35–36
    lipids, 36–37
    metabolic syndrome, 37–38
    mortality, 168, *168*
    obesity, 38–39
    overview, 29–30
    prostate cancer, 103
    risk of, 3, 17, *21*, 79, 103–104
    scope of the problem, 31
    stroke, 34–35
    treatment, 29–40
        weight gain, 111
        women, 39–40
Cardiovascular fitness, 81
Caucasians, 34
Centers for Disease Control and Prevention, 5
Cesarean delivery, 61
Chen, J., 116
Children and adolescents, 34
Chronic conditions, 9, 101–108
    in adults and children, *102*
    cancer survivors, 101–103
    hypertension, 103–104
    intellectual disabilities, 107
    multiple sclerosis (MS), 106
    osteoarthritis (OA), 103
    overview, 101
    spinal cord injuries (SCI), 106–107
    type 2 diabetes (T2DM), 105–106
Chronic diseases, **2**, 3–7; *see also* Diseases
    cardiovascular disease (CVD), 3–6
    risk of, 3
Chronic Obstructive Pulmonary Disease (COPD), 94
Cognition, 8, 124
Cognitive function, 8, 35, 72
    aspects of, 124
    brain health, 124–125
    older adults, 92–93
    in youth, 83
Cognitive impairment, 94
Cognitive reserve, 128–129
Colon cancer, 48, 71
Communicable diseases, 138
Communication environmental level, 180–182
    access to indoor/outdoor facilities, 182
    computer-tailored print interventions, 181
    interactive video games promoting active play
        or exercise, 182
    mobile phone programs, 181
    point of decision prompts, 182
    social media, 181
    telephone-assisted interventions, 181
    wearable activity monitors, 180–181
    web-based or internet-delivered interventions, 181
Community, 84
Community-based interventions, 177–180
Community organizations, 178–179
Community Preventive Sources Task Force, 179
Computer-tailored print interventions, 181
Coordinated Approach to Child Health
        (CATCH), 179
Coronary heart disease (CHD), 5, 30, 33, 67, 69,
        74, 165
Council on Lifestyle and Cardiometabolic
        Health, 17, 141
Council on Nutrition, Physical Activity and
        Metabolism, 17, 141
C-reactive protein (CRP), 117

D

Daily habits, 1; *see also* Physical activities/
    function
Da Qing Study, 7
Dementia, 3
Depression, 3, 8, 127; *see also* Anxiety
Diabetes, 6–7, 57–64; *see also* Cardiovascular
    disease (CVD); Obesity; Overweight;
    Prediabetes; Weight gain
  classifications of, 58
  risk of, 3
  type 1 diabetes (T1DM), 58, 59
  type 2 diabetes (T2DM), 17, *21*, 35, 37, 38,
    53, 57–58
  women's health, 67
Diabetes mellitus (DM), 38
Diabetes Prevention Program (DPP), 7, 62, 69
Diabetes Prevention study (DPS), 63
Diastolic blood pressure (DBP), 36, **36**, 104
Dietary Guidelines for Americans, 16
Diseases; *see also* Cancer(s); Cardiovascular
    disease (CVD); Chronic diseases;
    Obesity; Overweight; Weight gain
  Alzheimer disease (AD), 8, 72, 92
  communicable, 138
  heart, 39–40
  metabolic, 52–53
  myocardial infarction (MI), 69
  noncommunicable, 138
  Parkinson's disease, 94
  sudden cardiac death, 69, 75
Dishman, R., 178
Dose/dose response, 20–21
Downs Syndrome, 107
Dual-energy X-ray absorptiometry
    (DEXA), 144
Dyslipidemia, 38, 83

E

Educational resources, 142–43
Endometrial cancer, 48, 71
Energy intake, 115
Energy restriction, 113–114
Enjoyable experience, 161
Equipment, 162
Exercise, 17–18; *see also* Fitness; Physical
    activities/function
  adherence, 160
  intensity of, 19–20
  with others, 161
  routines, 162
  types of, 58–60
"Exercise Is Medicine (EIM)", 141,
    146–147

Exercise prescription, 144–146
  aerobic physical activity, 155–157
  balance, 159
  exercise adherence, 160
  flexibility, 158–159
  mind/body approaches, 160
  muscular fitness, 157–158
  overview, 153–154
  pre-participation screening, 154
  principles of, 155
  program, 161–162
  special populations, 160–161
  for special populations, 146
  workouts duration, 159

F

Fall prevention, older adults, 91–92
Finnish Diabetes Prevention Study, 7, 70
Fitness, 115–116; *see also* Exercise; Physical fitness
  evaluation, 143–144
  program, 162
Flexibility, 18, 158–159
Frailty, 94
Framingham Heart Study, 15, 104
Frequency, intensity, time and type (FITT), 147, 155

G

Gastric cancer, 48
Goodpaster, B., 114
Guide for Community Preventive Services, 180

H

Harvard Alumni Study, 112
Head and neck cancer, 48
Health, 1–12
  bone, 73
  breast, 71–72
  cost-effective mechanisms, 89
  outcomes, 115–116
  overview, 1–3
Health Belief Model (HBM), 175–176
Healthcare Providers Action Guide, 141
"Health-enhancing" physical activity, 49–50
Healthy People, 140
Heart disease, 39–40
Heart failure (HF), 38
Heart rate (HR), 81
Hematologic cancer, 48
High blood pressure, 6, 35, 83, 130
High-density lipoprotein-c (HDL-C), 117
Hip fracture, 94
Hispanics, 34
Household physical activity, 19
Hypertension, 35–36, 103–104, 116

I

Ideal cardiovascular health, 25
Impaired fasting glucose (IFG), 37, 38
Information and communication technologies
    (ICT), 180
Injury, 162
Insulin action, 60
Insulin-like growth factor (IGF-1), 93
Integrated behavior model (IBM), 176
Intellectual disabilities, 107
Intensity, 155
    absolute *vs.* relative, 19–20
    classifications, 19
    light activity, 20
    moderate activity, 19
    sedentary activity, 20
    vigorous activity, 19
Intention/Behavior Gap, 177
Interactive video games promoting active play or
    exercise, 182
Interleukin-6 (IL6), 117
Interventions
    adult, 182–183
    community-based, 177–180
    computer-tailored print, 181
    to reduce sedentary behavior, 182–183
    telephone-assisted, 181
    theory-based, 175–177
    web-based or internet-delivered, 181
    worksite, 182–183
    youth, 182

J

Jakicic, J., 114
Joint National Commission (JNC), 35
Journaling, 162

K

Kahn, R., 95

L

Lalonde, Marc, 15
Leisure time physical activity, 19
Lifestyle activity, 113
Lifestyle medicine, 1–12, 16–17, 138, 153
Lifestyle Medicine (Blackwell Science), 1, 175
Lifestyle Medicine Education Collaborative
    (LMEd), 143
Light intensity activity, 20
Lipid Research Clinic Study, 116
Lipids, 36–37, 79
Look AHEAD Study, 116
Low-density lipoprotein cholesterol (LDL-C), 36–37

Low-density lipoproteins (LDL), 117
Low levels of high-density cholesterol (HDL-C),
    36–37
Lung cancer, 48, 71

M

Major depressive disorders (MDD), 127
Measuring physical activity, 21–22
Menopause, 73
Menstrual dysfunction, 75
Metabolic disease, 52–53
Metabolic equivalents (MET), 19, 145, **145**
Metabolic Syndrome (METS), 6–7, 17, 37–38,
    57–64, 111
Mexican Americans, 34
Mild cognitive impairment (MCI), 92
Mind/body activities, 19
Mind/body approaches, 160
Minimizing exertion, 62
Mobile phone programs, 181
Moderate intensity physical activity, 19, 22, 31, 33
Moderate physical activity, 145
Moderate to vigorous physical activity (MVPA),
    3, 5, *6*, *23*, *32*, 80–81, 83, *139*, *166*,
    167, *168*, 169–170, 178
Monitoring physical activity, 22
Multiple sclerosis (MS), 106
Muscle strengthening activities, 18
Muscular fitness, 81, 157–158
Musculoskeletal injuries, 75
Myocardial infarction (MI), 31, 39, 69

N

National Cholesterol Education Program (NCEP), 37
National Comprehensive Cancer Network, 49
National Health and Nutrition Examination
    Survey (NHANES), 38, 112
National Health Interviews Survey, 90
National Heart, Lung and Blood Institute
    (NHLBI), 37
National Highway Traffic Safety Administration, 128
National Institute of Health (NIH), 7
National Physical Activity Plan, 182
Non-communicable diseases (NCD), 138, 141
Nonprofit organizations, 178–179
Nurse Delivered Programs, 180
Nurses' Health Study, 70–71, 73

O

Obesity, 50, 60; *see also* Cardiovascular
    disease (CVD); Diabetes; Overweight;
    Weight gain
    physical activities, 7–8, 17, 111–117
    women's health, 67

Obstructive sleep apnea (OSA), 128
Occupational physical activity, 19, 21
Older adults, 9, 17, 34, 89–97
    cognitive function, 92–93
    fall prevention, 91–92
    overview, 89–90
    reducing age associated sarcopenia, 93
    risk of fracture, 91, *92*
    successful aging, 95–96
One-mile Walk Test, 154
Optimal brain health, 25–26, 129–130;
        see also Brain health
"Optimizing Brain Health," 8
Osteoarthritis (OA), 9, 103
Osteoporosis, 73, 94; *see also* Brain health
Ovarian cancer, 49, 71
Overcoming sedentary behavior, 9, 165–170
Overweight, 38, 50; *see also* Cardiovascular
        disease (CVD); Diabetes; Diseases;
        Obesity; Weight gain

P

Pancreatic cancer, 49
Parkinson's disease, 94
Physical activities/function, 1–12;
        see also Exercise
    adherence, 51–52
    adverse events, 62
    aerobic, 18, 59
    anaerobic, 18
    balance training, 18
    benefits, 6, 31, 59
    body composition, 74
    body position, 19
    bone strengthening activities, 18
    brain health, 8, 35, 123–131
    cancer, 18, 45–54
    in cancer prevention, 46–48
    cardiovascular disease (CVD), 29–40, *105*
    categorization of, 22
    chronic diseases, **2**, 3–7
    clinical recommendations, **51**
    cognition, 8, 123–131
    concepts, 15–27
    coronary heart disease (CHD), 69
    devices to measure, 21–22
    diabetes, 6–7, 57–64
    domains of, 19
    dose of, 20–21
    evaluating patients for, 10
    exercise, 17–18
    flexibility training, 18
    food and insulin management with, 61
    "health-enhancing," 49–50
    for healthy individuals, 10
    household, 19

in individuals with chronic conditions, 9, 101–108
    insulin action and, 60
    intensity of, 19–20
    leisure time, 19
    lifestyle medicine and, 16–17
    lipids and, 37
    measurements, 21–22
    metabolic syndrome, 6–7, 57–64
    minimizing exertion, 62
    moderate, 22
    moderate-intensity, 19, 22, 31
    moderate *vs.* vigorous, 3, 5, *6*, *23*, *32*
    monitoring, 22
    muscle strengthening activities, 18
    obesity, 7–8, 50, 60, 111–117
    occupational, 19
    older adults, 9, 89–97, 93–95
    organizations, **2**
    overcoming sedentary behavior, 9
    physicians' role, 3, 10, 137–149
    physical fitness *vs.,* 22–24, *24*, 33
    in prediabetes, 6–7, 57–64, 62–63
    in pregnancy, 7, 61–62
    professional organizations, 141–142
    promotion of, 26–27, 173–183
    public health considerations, 10
    Qigong, 19
    recommendations, **2**, 33–34
    research, 53
    resistance exercise, 59
    risks of, 75
    safety during, 26
    for special populations, 10
    steps in promoting, 10–11
    strategies for, 52
    strong evidence of protective effects,
        cancer, 48–49
    Tai Chi, 19
    transportation, 19
    type 2 diabetes (T2DM), 69–70
    types of, 18–19, 58–60
    vigorous intensity, 19, 22, 33
    volume, 20–21
    weight gain, 7–8, 111–117
    women's health, 7, 67–76
    yoga, 19
    youth, 8, 79–85
Physical activity bouts, duration, 113
Physical Activity Guidelines Advisory (PAGA)
        Committee Report, 2, 3, **4–5**, 5, 8, 11,
        16, 17, 24, 30–31, 46, 48, 59, 67, 68,
        70, 74, 79–80, 90, 103, 111, 124, 153
Physical activity program, 162
Physical Activity Readiness Questionnaire (PAR
        Q), 154
Physical fitness; *see also* Fitness
        across the lifespan, 24–25

components of, 24
defined, 22, 143
ideal cardiovascular health, 25
physical activities *vs.*, 22–24, *24*, 33
tests of, 33
Physician(s), 3, 10, 137–149
educational resources, 142–143
exercise prescription, 144–146
fitness evaluation, 143–144
lifestyle medicine, 138
overview, 137–138
promotion and involvement of, 138–140
rationale for, 142
recommendations for physical activity, 140, 141
resources, 148
as a role model, 147–148
utilizing experts, 147
wish to get started, 146–147
Planned Behavior and Integrated Behavior
    Model, 176
Point of decision prompts, 182
Positive psychology, 177
Positron emission tomography (PET), 125, 127
Prediabetes, 6–7, 57–64; *see also* Diabetes
    classifications of, 58
    physical activities in, 6–7, 62–63
    types of, 58
Preeclampsia, 61
Pre-exercise health screening and evaluation, 61
Pregnancy, 7, 61–62
    post-partum and, 72–73
    women's health, 72–73
Pre-participation screening, 154
Primary cancer prevention, 46–47
Primary care physicians, 39
Primary care settings, 180
Primordial prevention, 25
Prochaska, J., 176
Professional organizations, 141–142
Program of regular physical activity, 161–162
Promotion of physical activities, 173–183
    communication environmental level, 180–182
    community-based interventions, 177–180
    conceptual framework for factors influencing,
        173–174
    individual level, 174–175
    interventions to reduce sedentary behavior,
        182–183
    overview, 173
    social ecological framework, *174*
    theory-based interventions, 175–177
Prostate cancer, 49, 103
Protocol, *see specific protocol*
Public health, 96
    considerations, 10
    impacts, 95, 170
Public recreation facilities, 179

Q

Qigong, 19, 90
Quality of Life (QoL), 123, 125–126, 130

R

Randomized controlled trial (RCT), 73, 90, 91
Rankinen, T., 116
Realistic goals, 162
Rectal cancer, 49
Registered Clinical Exercise Physiologist
    (RCEP), 147
Renal cancer, 48
Resistance exercise, 59, 112
Resting metabolic rate (RMR), 115
Reward yourself, 162
Richmond, J., 15, 140
Rippe Lifestyle Institute (RLI), 1, 137, 153–154, 156
Rowe, J., 95

S

San Diego County, 179
Sarcopenia, 93
School(s), 83–84, 177–178
School Health Policies and Practices Study, 83
Secondary cancer prevention, 47
Sedentary activity, 20
Sedentary behavior, 9, 59–60, 113; *see also*
        Overcoming sedentary behavior
    all-cause mortality, 165–168, *166*, *167*
    cancers and, 50, 169
    cardiovascular disease (CVD) mortality,
        168, *168*
    defined, 19, 165
    moderate to vigorous physical activity
        (MVPA), *166*, *167*, *168*, 169–170
    overcoming, 9, 165–170
    overview, 165
    public health impact, 170
    type 2 diabetes (T2DM), 169
    weight status, 169
    youth, 82–83
Self-efficacy, 115, 176
Short Form Health Survey (SF-36), 90, 125
"Simple 7," 30
Single Leg Stand Test, 159
Sleep, 127–128
Social Cognitive Theory (SCT), 176–177
Spinal cord injuries (SCI), 106–107
Stanford University, 154
Stroke, 34–35, 95, 124
Successful aging, 89, 95–96
Systolic blood pressure (SBP), 35, **36**, 104, 116
Systolic Blood Pressure Intervention Trial
    (SPRINT), 35

T

Tai Chi, 19, 59, 90
Telephone-assisted interventions, 181
Tertiary cancer treatment, 47–48
Theory-based interventions, 175–177
Theory of Planned Behavior (TPB), 176
Theory of Reasoned Action (TRA), 176
Thyroid cancer, 49
Time, 155
Tissue necrosis factor α(TNFα), 117
Total cholesterol (TC), 36
Transient Ischemic Attacks (TIA), 35
Transportation physical activity, 19
Trans Theoretical Model (TTM), 176
Triglycerides (TG), 36
Type, 155
Type 1 diabetes (T1DM), 58, 59, 61
Type 2 diabetes (T2DM), 17, *21*, 35, 37, 38, 53,
        57–58, 61, 63, 74, 80, 165, 169
    women's health, 67, 69–70

U

United States, 3, 7–8, 22, 30, 35, 39, 45–46, 79
U.S. National Activity Plan, 141
U.S. National Cancer Institute, 101
U.S. National Health and Nutrition Examination
        Survey (NHANES), 9, 165
U.S. National Physical Activity Program, 146, 154

V

Vigorous intensity physical activities, 19
Visual impairments, 95
Volume, physical activity, 20–21

W

Walking, 113, 156–157
Wearable activity monitors, 180–181
Web-based or internet-delivered interventions,
        181
Weight control, 70
Weight gain, 7–8, 111–117; *see also*
        Cardiovascular disease (CVD);
        Diabetes; Obesity; Overweight
    energy expenditure, 115
    factors influencing adherence, 115
    fitness, 115–116
    health outcomes, 115–116
    METS, 111

    overview, 111
    prevention of, 111–112
    type 2 diabetes (T2DM), 111
Weight loss, 112–114
    variability, 114–115
Weight status, 169
White, Paul Dudley, 15
Wing, R., 114, 116
Women, 39–40, 67–76
    all-cause mortality, 68
    body composition, 74
    bone health/osteoporosis, 73
    brain health/cognitive function, 72
    breast health, 71–72
    cancers, 70–71
    coronary heart disease (CHD), 69
    diabetes, 67
    menopause, 73
    obesity, 67
    overview, 67–68
    pregnancy and post-partum, 72–73
    risks of physical activity, 75
    sports, 74–75
    type 2 diabetes (T2DM), 67, 69–70
    weight control, 70
Women's Health Initiative Observational Study, 69
Workouts duration, exercise prescription, 159
Worksites, 178
    interventions, 182–183
World Cancer Research Fund International, 46, 70
World Health Organization (WHO), 138

Y

Yoga, 19, 90
Youth, 8, 79–85
    academic achievement, 83
    adiposity, 81–82
    body weight, 81–82
    bone health, 82
    cardiometabolic health, 80–81
    cardiovascular fitness, 81
    cognitive function, 83
    community, 84
    family, 83–84
    government strategies, 83–84
    health, 82–83
    interventions, 182
    muscular fitness, 81
    overview, 79–80
    school, 83–84
    sedentary behavior, 82–83